CW01301146

BODY WISDOM

An Easy Guide to Maintaining a Comfortable (and good looking) Body

Jackie Wright

Drawings by Sandy Morris

authorHOUSE®

AuthorHouse™ UK Ltd.
500 Avebury Boulevard
Central Milton Keynes, MK9 2BE
www.authorhouse.co.uk
Phone: 08001974150

©2010 Jackie Wright. All rights reserved.

No part of this book may be reproduced, stored in a retrieval system, or transmitted by any means without the written permission of the author.

First published by AuthorHouse   10/13/2010

ISBN: 978-1-4520-8157-1 (sc)

This book is printed on acid-free paper.

Contents

Chapter 1. Body Systems   1

  Circulation - The Importance of Blood   1
  Lubrication – how to oil the joints.   2
  Joints   4
  Muscles, Tendons and Ligaments.   5
  Nerves   7

Chapter 2. A Body Survey   8

  Feet to Hips   8
    Feet   8
    Ankles   11
    Knees   12
    Hips   15
  Hands to Shoulders   16
    Hands   16
    The Wrist.   18
    Elbows   20
    Shoulders   21
  The Spine   24
    The Neck / Cervical Spine   25
    Thoracic Spine   27
    Lumbar Spine   27
    Sacro-Iliac joint: 32

Chapter 3. Physical Skills for Easy Living.   33

  Posture   33
  Tension   39
    Good stress and bad stress   39
    Relaxation Techniques   41
  Stretching   43
    Why Stretch   43
    When and How to Stretch   44

Individual Stretches	**45**
Calf muscles:	45
Thigh muscles – Quadriceps:	46
Hamstrings	47
Back muscles	48
Upper back	48
Neck	50
Shoulders	50
Jaw	50
Forearms	51
Hands	51
Hip and shoulder rotation	51
Spinal rotation	52
Strength and Control	**52**
The deep stomach muscles	53
The shoulder-blades	53
Pelvic Floor muscles:	53
Balance	**54**

Chapter 4. Activities in daily life — 57

In Praise of Walking	**57**
Household Tips	**60**
Gardening Tips	**62**
Driving Tips	**63**
Occupations	**64**
Sedentary jobs e.g. at Computers.	64
Hard physical jobs.	65
Landscape Gardeners	65
Carpet layers.	66
Forklift Drivers.	67
Carers	67
Leisure Activities	**68**
Running for Amateurs	68
Cycling.	69
Swimming and Aqua-aerobics.	69
Dancing / Exercises to music.	70
Yoga.	70

Chapter 5. Common Problems — 71

- 'Aches and Pains' — 71
- Arthritis. — 72
- Illness — 74
- Injury — 74
  - Broken bones: — 74
  - Torn muscles: — 75
  - Torn or sprained tendons and ligaments: — 75
- Breathlessness. — 75

Chapter 6. Keeping Old Age at Bay — 77

- Danger – Beware! — 78
- Summing up — 79
- Suggested Daily Routine — 80

Acknowledgements.

Many thanks to Nicholas for his patience, his instructive ideas and his editing.

Thanks also to my colleagues Bridget King and Alison Garner for checking the facts in this book, and to Jenny James for her many useful comments.

The logistics for the artist, being either in France or Nepal, have sometimes been challenging. Thank you Sandy!

Introduction

Pain alters our lives. Comfort, ease of movement, flexibility, co-ordination, balance, strength, sleep – all can be affected. Even our family and social life can change, with pain causing fatigue, loss of confidence, irritability, depression. We give little thought to our bodies – until something goes wrong. Often we are bewildered by this pain – where has it come from; what did I do? Anxiety may set in. Is it cancer, is it arthritis, am I getting old? Approximately 20% of visits to GPs are because of musculo-skeletal pain - pain affecting joints and muscles - yet very often this is due to a relatively simple problem, which could have been avoided – if only we had known how. Pain so often is unnecessary.

Yes, prevention **is** better than cure. None of us would let a day go by without cleaning our teeth. It has become a habit because no one likes toothache and we want our teeth to look good when we smile. We may still get toothache but far less frequently than if we paid no attention to our teeth. But what about the rest of our body? That can ache too and look less good than it should. Perhaps we don't do any maintenance or preventative work on the body because we don't really know what to do that is simple, that can fit into our normal day, that becomes a habit - like cleaning our teeth.

This book has come about because over the years of working as a physiotherapist the people who have come to me have said time and time again: "if only I had known that before. Why didn't anyone tell me?" It's a book to dip into, or to use to refer to a section that interests you. There is some general information about how the body works There is a section on each part of the body. There are some "maintenance tips" – and a few warnings. It will NOT answer all health problems. It is NOT in place of going to your doctor if you are in a great deal of pain or having other unusual symptoms.

I hope you will find that the advice given is simple common-sense, so that you end up saying: "why didn't I think of that before?"

The message of the book is: if you are in good health it pays huge dividends to maintain this, easily and habitually, by following these simple rules:-

Think tall – Relax – 'Wriggle' – Stretch – Keep active.

This book will explain why these are important and how to make them part of your everyday life.

If you are not in good health, or are unfit, or been injured, or have stiffened up, it may take a bit of time and effort to regain a body that you enjoy and can live with comfortably and confidently - but it is time well spent. The rewards are great.

Living creatures have developed over millions of years. They have become very efficient at what they need to do for survival, to keep the species going. Humans, and presumably other long-lived creatures such as elephants and tortoises, have developed ways of maintaining the body tissue so that it keeps working efficiently for many years. Our cells are continually renewing themselves.

Without us realising it we have a change of skin, muscle, bone etc. on a regular basis. This process also helps tissue to heal if it has been damaged. But we are living longer, thanks to better sanitation, nutrition, and medical intervention. And the natural renewal process slows down after half a century or so – bone may become less strong, muscle less elastic, blood vessels less pliable, cartilage less smooth and protective, especially if we do nothing to maintain them. A history of accidents, major and minor, throughout our lives will mean there are areas of scar-tissue and if we don't keep this supple we will stiffen up and so become more susceptible to painful strains.

Fortunately there are some simple things we can do to help our bodies remain comfortable. I have met several people in their eighties and nineties who are living active lives – this is the key - and move around with ease and confidence, without discomfort. I have also seen many who are decades younger who already feel old, who are unable to get out of a chair easily, who can't get comfortable at night, who have lost confidence in their body's abilities. Some have inherited a problem but many have allowed their bodies to deteriorate. It is amazing what a difference it can make to develop an awareness of how the body works, and to listen to what it is telling you.

Chapter 1.
Body Systems

Circulation - The Importance of Blood

Blood brings oxygen and nutrition to all parts of the body. Some parts, that are working especially hard, need a greater supply. For example, our brains are very demanding. So are the muscles that keep us upright and moving around. If we are anaemic for any reason we feel tired and weak. If we have low blood pressure we may at first feel dizzy and faint when we stand up suddenly – not enough blood has reached the brain so it is unable to function fully.

Blood is pumped around the body by the heart but also by the action of other muscles. When muscles are active blood is pumped around the body efficiently and the tissues are well supplied; our skin looks good, we feel good, we move well. Muscles function better when they are used often. It is activity which keeps them strong. And this is also true of the heart, as it too is a muscle. When we are inactive, although the heart continues working it is not being supported by the other muscle pumps. The supply of oxygen and nutrients is less good so tissues are starved. They may complain by aching. We may feel sluggish and every activity, even thought, may become more of an effort.

Another important role of our circulation is to remove the waste products produced by muscle work. If these waste products (Lactic Acid etc.) remain in the tissues they can become very tender - as you might expect from acid.

Our temperature control is also dependent on our circulation – you know how cold you can get if you sit still for long.

Blood plays a vital contribution in the healing process. It transports the necessary ingredients for healing of the damaged part to occur. Tissues with good circulation heal faster.

Common sense therefore tells us that being active is 'good' for us and being inactive is 'bad'.

Lubrication – how to oil the joints.

Frequently patients have told me how surprised they are at the good results they get from the very gentle, easy exercises I have taught them, which they actually enjoy doing! "Shouldn't exercises be painful?" I am often asked. "Surely there is no gain without pain?" or "My partner tells me I should be working harder. These silly little exercises can't possibly be doing anything!" But in fact they are, and this is why:

All the moving parts of a machine need oil to keep them working smoothly. This is true of our moving parts too, especially our joints. Rather than having to squirt in WD40 (a spray-lubricant), we have an in-built lubricating mechanism. As we move our joints, however gently, oil (synovial fluid) is pumped into the joint. When we are not moving the oil begins to dry out. This is why many people feel stiff after they have been sitting or lying still for any length of time. Perhaps this is more obvious as we get older – or is it simply that we don't move so much? It is a simple matter to get the circulation flowing and pump oil into the joints. We can do this by moving about / 'wriggling' before we get out of bed in the morning and if we are sitting for any length of time. Here are some examples of what I call 'wriggling', but once you get a feel for it you can invent your own. The important thing is that these movements should be natural, easy, comfortable (and that means no pain) and smooth. They require no effort and can be done in any position and at any time. It only takes a few repetitions to get that oil flowing. The following 'wriggles' are especially good for the spine:

- When sitting – at a desk, watching a film, while driving – with your feet on the floor, or on the pedals (at a safe moment), keep your feet still but gently slide one knee forward as the other slides back. Repeat smoothly and easily several times.
- Lying with your knees bent – tilt your pelvis so that your low back flattens. Then tilt it in the other direction so that your back

arches. Rock up and down several times, making the movement slower and smaller until it feels absolutely comfortable – and repeat at this level. The less muscle tension you use the better. You may find it helps to breathe in as you arch your back and breathe out as it flattens. Once you can feel how to do this movement in lying, you will also be able to do it in sitting or standing – and it does wonders for the back.

- Lying on your back with your knees bent - rock your knees to one side and roll your head to the other. This is a lovely movement that lubricates the whole spine – and it should feel pleasurable. Remember not to put any effort into the movement, only going as far as feels comfortable. It should feel completely natural and effortless. In fact it is how the spine moves as we walk.

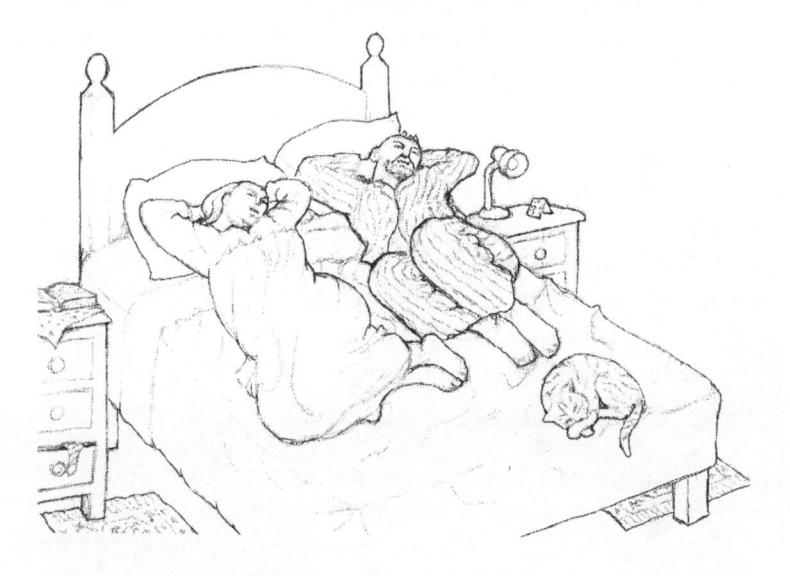

- Move your shoulders up and down; one up as the other moves down. Check that they move smoothly, without any jerkiness. If they continue to be jerky try doing it in the bath, as the support of the water allows them to move more smoothly, and you will be able to feel how easy it should be.

A wonderful lubricating exercise is walking - as long as we walk with good posture, are relaxed, and allow our legs and arms to swing easily.

> When a number of patients with Back pain are referred for Physiotherapy I often invite them to attend a Back Advice Group while waiting for their individual appointment. As well as general advice I teach them how to do these sort of movements. Frequently when then invited for an individual appointment people have said "Now that I know how to 'wriggle' my back pain has gone away. I can't believe something so simple could work!"

Joints

The ends of the bones where they meet each other and form a joint are shaped according to their function. The joints that bear our weight need to be strong and stable with broad surfaces. The ones that need to be flexible, such as the shoulder, have shallower, less stable surfaces to permit a wide range of movements. The bone ends are covered with a silky-smooth, strong coating of cartilage. Some joints have extra cartilage between the bone ends which acts as a cushion or shock-absorber, e.g. the knees, the jaw, between each vertebra. Joints move more easily if there is space between the bone ends. There is naturally some space there but this will be reduced if we over-tension the muscles around the joint or subject them to too much weight. Lubrication, *(see above)* assists the smooth movement.
Joints are held together by ligaments and controlled by muscles.

> A lady came to see me complaining of a stiff, painful neck and terrible grating sounds whenever she turned her head. When I gently took the weight of her head so that the joints lifted off each other the pain disappeared. When she then kept that feeling of space and turned her head there was no grating. Once she knew how to do that – and no longer feared that she had 'crumbling bones' – her movement improved, the pain and the grating ceased – unless she tensed up again. But now she understood the reason and was able to control it.

Joints can move in a variety of directions to permit the variety of activities that we need – small sideways or rotation movements, for example to allow us to walk on rough, uneven surfaces. If we lose these, activities become more difficult, less co-ordinated, more uncomfortable. It is important to retain full range movement in all directions. If you feel that a joint is becoming even a little stiff keep nudging at that stiffness until it goes away.

Muscles, Tendons and Ligaments.

Muscles - there are about 700 muscles, of different sizes and shapes depending on their function. Generally the deep muscles, close to the joints, are short and act as protection to the joint, holding it in a correct position, making minor adjustments to its position as required by our changes in posture, and assisting our balance. They are therefore active most of the time and so are designed to work at a low level for long periods.

The superficial muscles tend to be longer and often cross two or more joints. This is so that neighbouring joints work efficiently together. When we are walking we want our hips and knees and ankles to be co-ordinated. When reaching for something all the joints of our arm need to work together. So these long muscles are our action muscles. They work when they have a job to do and should relax when that action is complete. This contraction / relaxation leads to a pumping effect which helps the circulation of the blood.

Muscles are elastic and so their length can alter. With most actions they shorten as they are activated. When they relax they should return to their longer, resting length. If they have worked hard for a long period of time they may remain shorter than they should. It is therefore a good idea to stretch them back to their normal resting length after activities such as gardening, sport, a long walk. As they act as guy ropes, holding our bodies in position, they need to be the correct length. What would your tent look like if one guy rope was shorter than the others? Sometimes you can see this imbalance in people who have done a lot of weight lifting, if they have built up one group of muscles more than the opposing ones and not stretched afterwards.

If we continue holding tension in the superficial muscles they may take over from the deep muscles – but not as efficiently. The deep ones may then reduce their activity and so become weaker. This is particularly common in the muscles around the spine and shoulders and can lead to incorrect posture and back and neck ache.

Muscles love to be active; this is what keeps them strong and healthy. If they are not used they become weaker and less efficient and this leads to more strain on the body.

Tendons and Ligaments - muscle tissue becomes tougher and less elastic where it attaches to bone. This part of a muscle is called a tendon and they vary in length and strength depending on their function. Some are long and thin, like those going to our fingers. Some are shorter and stronger, like those needed to support the body e.g. the Achilles tendon, which attaches the calf muscles to the heel bone.

Ligaments tie the bones together, and are much less elastic than muscle tissue, in order to keep the joints stable. Both ligaments and tendons, because they have less "give", are more likely to be sprained or torn when put under sudden pressure or when trying to support too much weight. They also do not have a good blood supply and so can take longer to heal when damaged.

Some people have lax ligaments; they are "hypermobile". They can move their joints into extreme positions, such as bending their thumb back onto their forearm. They are often very good at gymnastics because they are so flexible. But they are more likely to strain their joints. If their short, supportive muscles are strong this is less of a problem. Those muscles, in some cases, can also take the place of ligaments that have been torn – but it may take some hard work.

> A friend who was a very keen mountain-climber was upset that his problem knee wouldn't allow him to climb any more. He had torn the ligaments in an accident. I suggested he try to build up the muscles around the knee by standing on that leg and beginning to do a squat. At first he could only bend and control the knee a few degrees but he was keen and persisted. Eventually he was able to do a full squat, standing on the one leg – and found he was able to climb again. Ten years later he is still climbing regularly.

Nerves

Nerves are our lines of communication. Messages are sent along them all over the body. They come from the brain, down the spinal cord and out to each muscle, telling them what action to perform. Others work in the other direction, bringing sensory messages from skin, joints, muscles, eyes, ears, nose, mouth, internal organ, - to the brain. This constant, complex system allows us to function effectively and creatively in this infinitely varied world. We develop **habits** of thought and movement by repetition – quick routes along nerves, familiarity in muscles - which make those thoughts and actions even easier, so we don't have to think how to do them. With practice we can become amazingly skilled at complex activities. Sometimes, however, habits such as poor posture or biting our nails, are not so useful to us. With persistence, we can change to a better habit - once we understand what that is.

Of course nerves are sensitive structures. If they are irritated we may feel strange sensations such as 'pins and needles' or pain of various kinds. If they are compressed, messages will be blocked and then the area will feel numb or a muscle will not respond. Most of us have slept on an arm, compressing the nerve at the elbow, and woken with a 'dead' hand. Once the pressure is relieved and we move the hand, it tingles and then returns to normal. But if the irritation or pressure remains so does that unnatural sensation. Nerves supply particular areas of the body and specific muscles and that information can help to identify where the problem comes from. Once you know that, and if you can then create more space for the nerve at that point, then it can start to function properly again. It may however take some time for the nerve to fully heal if it has been damaged. They can become scarred, like any healing tissue, and that may need to be stretched. You would need advice from a physiotherapist on how to do that without irritating the nerve.

The sensation of pain travels along nerves. It can be a useful message telling us, for example, to remove a hand from a hot surface or to move out of an uncomfortable position. We are wise to respond to this message. The cause of the pain is obvious when we have had an accident: a cut, a broken bone, damaged tissue. Deep internal pain is often difficult to identify and requires further investigation.

Sometimes nerves become so used to sending pain messages that they continue doing so for no valid reason – a pain 'habit'. They may need to be taught how to get out of this distressing habit by someone experienced in the management of chronic pain.

Chapter 2.
A Body Survey

__Feet to Hips__

Feet

    Feet must be **supple** in order to accept uneven ground and cushion the impact when we walk or run. There are 28 bones in a foot and they should all move on each other. That's easy: wriggle your toes, spread them wide, move your foot and ankle in all directions.

    Feet must be **strong** in order to bear your weight and to be able to push you forward when walking or running. But how can 28 little bones be strong? Large buildings, like churches, have arches to support them because an arch gives strong support. Feet need arches for strength too but they have to be mobile ones. The main arch is on the inner side of your foot – the instep. This arch flattens as weight goes onto it, to soften the impact throughout the body, but immediately the strong muscles of the lower leg should pull up the instep and this will lock the bones into a sturdy arch.

Some people seem to inherit very flat feet and there doesn't seem to be much they can do about it, other than keep the muscles strong and wear good, supportive shoes and insoles.

Others inherit very high arches, which are often stiff. Not such good shock-absorbers, so it pays to try to keep them as supple as possible and perhaps wear shock-absorbing insoles.

Many people have **flat feet** because they have never strengthened the necessary muscles, perhaps because they have a sedentary job. It's never too late to do so, and it is so worthwhile, because flat feet can lead to twisted ankles, knees, hips, back. Over time this can cause damage to the cartilage of those joints.

Painful feet are very disabling. Another joint frequently affected is the big toe. A twisting pressure onto it - because of the flattened arch - can push it in, cause a bunion, and even distort the other toes, (so can tight shoes of course). If it stiffens or is fixed surgically we lose the normal push-off. This will affect our rhythm of walking and therefore the whole body.

How do we strengthen feet?
- Start by sitting with your feet flat on the ground. Pull up your instep – it's only a small movement – not by crinkling up your toes but by tensioning the muscles either side of your lower leg. Keep all your toes on the ground while you do this. Then relax. Repeat several times.
- Every time you go to stand up, pull up the arches first, so that your feet take your weight without rolling in. If your knees are directly over your toes, rather than falling in towards each other, your arches are probably working well.
- Do the arch exercise in standing as well. They have to work harder when they are taking your weight.
- Make them work harder still by going up on your toes and

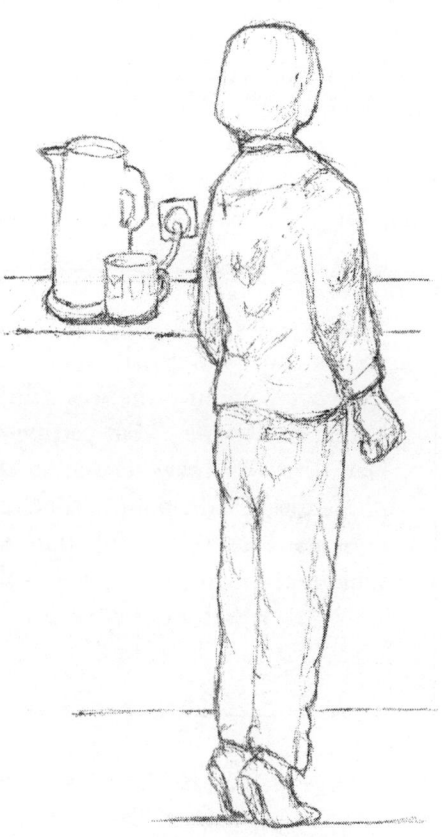

really pulling up your insteps. You could do a few while waiting for the kettle to boil.
- As you walk push off with your Big Toe; that's why it is big. Its job is to push off, with your feet in a straight line, and this will trigger the muscles that create the arch.
- Don't walk with your feet pointing out, like a duck. Your feet will flatten, your big toe will be pushed in, you will strain the inside of your ankles and knees, your hip muscles will work incorrectly and you will compress your low back. Sounds awful! It is unlikely you will notice any symptoms for many years – but then, perhaps suddenly, something will start to complain.

Notice the way other people walk – it can become a fascinating study!

The foot is supported by strong tissue called the Plantar Fascia. This can become strained and inflamed – Plantar Fasciitis – and can be very painful, especially when you first take weight on it in the morning. You may be able to ease this by having a comfortable, supportive insole, carefully stretching it (see p. 46) and massaging it.

> A very active man in his late fifties asked for advice. He had always run, played golf, skiied etc. but now the bottom of his feet were so painful he was thinking he would have to give up his active lifestyle. "I'm getting old. It's awful". Certainly his feet were extremely tender, so that he yelled when they were pressed at certain points. But once he knew how to give local massage to those painful spots, stretched, and bought himself some appropriate insoles, he was able eventually to return to those activities. It was a great relief to him that his active life was not over. Not so old after all!

There is a fat pad under the heel to cushion the thousands of little impacts upon it. As we get older this can thin out and if it does become painful we can protect it by a nice, comfortable gel pad under the heel. Avoid hard-soled shoes. Listen as your heel hits the ground – and walk softly.

Feet are precious. If they become stiff and painful it can affect your whole body. You are unable to move around with ease and this can become very tiring and frustrating. Life becomes hard. So it pays to look after them, keeping them supple and strong.

They love to be massaged!

And wear good shoes for the work they have to do. This mainly means enough room for the toes and firm support under the instep – especially when running or hiking. Please do them up too – teenagers often seem to walk around with their shoes undone– and this will cause all sorts of bad habits for the hips and feet. I find walking around shops or museums, on hard surfaces, can be extremely tiring and a good pair of shoes can make all the difference.

Ankles

The ankle joint consists of one of the bones of the foot, the Talus, held between the two bones of your lower leg, the Tibia and Fibula, and held together by strong ligaments Movement between these three bones should, of course, be smooth but that is less likely if the foot is not in alignment – most likely to occur if feet are flat or turned out.

If you keep spraining it check the following:
- ▶ Have you full movement in the ankle joint? Compare it to the other one.
  If not, exercise it to regain full movement.
- ▶ Are your calf muscles tight? These muscles can become tight if you usually wear high heels or if you sit most of the time.
  If they are, stretch them regularly. (see p. 45)
- ▶ Is it strong? Can you stand on one leg and go up on your toes? Hold on to something if necessary.
  If not, practice doing that until you can do it easily. Walk regularly.
- ▶ Is your heel bone, the Calcaneum, square on the ground or does it tilt? Is the tendon which joins onto it, the Achilles tendon, straight or curved? Ask someone to have a look. If the bone is tilted and the tendon curved (this is quite common) and you are having problems, a wedge- shaped insole to counteract the tilt may help. Also check the advice on Flat feet.
- ▶ Can you balance on one leg – steady – and close your eyes? Can you count up to ten while doing this? You are much more likely to keep spraining your ankle if you can't. Practice doing this – safely –until you can do it easily.

> A keen, young footballer came with a swollen, painful ankle. He couldn't understand why he had sprained it so easily. It turned out that he had severely sprained it twice before. He had regained full movement and strength, but no-one had suggested he needed to balance on one leg with his eyes closed! When he tried to do this, he couldn't. Too wobbly. But he started practising and quite quickly mastered it. He was able to play football with no further sprains.

Calf muscles need to work regularly. They are an important assistant to the heart, pumping blood and other fluids up the legs. One of the reasons for swollen ankles is that the calf muscles are not sufficiently active. How do we use them? Simply by walking, or more strongly by running, with a good push-off. They won't work as well if the feet are turned out a lot or if you are not using that Big toe. If you can't go out for a walk you could do some ballet exercises! Go up on your toes several times. That will work the calf muscles. Or at least pump your feet up and down and circle them round several times while you are sitting or lying.

Remember to give them a nice, slow stretch if they have worked hard, to regain their full resting length. I've often found that people who suffer from **cramp** or **restless legs** benefit from stretching them regularly, especially just before going to bed. (see p. 45)

Knees

What a lot of hard work they have to do! That's why the knee joint is immensely strong, with plenty of cushioning and many strong muscles to do the work. They are designed to work and they like it. They are not so happy when they sit still for a long time. We think of it as a hinge joint i.e. it opens and closes / straightens and bends, which it is doing all the time as we walk, go up and down stairs, go from sitting to standing etc. But it also has to be able to adjust to rough ground and take all sorts of twisting strains – especially if you play football.

Try sitting up on a high surface so that your feet are not touching the ground. Let your legs dangle. Swing them loosely. Then swing them in circles and you will discover quite a lot of extra movement. By the way, knees love this sort of exercise so, if you find they ache, sit and swing for a few minutes and they may well feel happier.

If you find it hard to go downstairs in the morning, because your knees feel stiff and unsafe, sit on the edge of the bed and swing them a few times.

Weight-bearing twisting activities do place a great strain on the joint and all the structures around it. So when you go to stand up, or are going up or down steps, check that your knees point directly over your feet, not inwards, and that the arches of your feet are slightly raised. Also check that your shoes aren't badly worn down on one side of the heel.

Like all joints knees find it a strain to carry more weight than they are designed for. The force through the leg we are standing on and pushing off with, as the other leg is swinging through, has been calculated as approximately FOUR times our body weight. Many people who have knee pain and are over-weight find the pain is greatly relieved when they lose a couple of stone. You are far less likely to need a knee replacement if you are not over-weight.

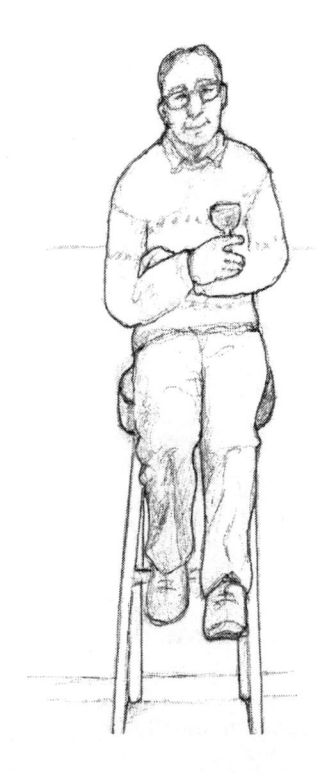

If the muscles around the knee are strong they protect the joint and it can tolerate more.

If they are not strong, perhaps because you don't walk much or have been unable to walk recently, the joint will have less protection. So, keep walking! Use your common sense about how far you can go, especially if you have not been walking much recently, but try to walk most days. Using a stick, in the **opposite** hand to the problem knee, can take about 20% of body weight.

You can do exercises too. It is especially important to be able to fully straighten your knee. If you can't and are walking with the knees bent you will put far more strain on the muscles and the joints. Try sitting straight on a firm chair. Now straighten one knee, lifting your lower leg up, and brace your thigh muscle. Check if the knee is completely straight. Can you hold it there for the count of ten? Can you lower it smoothly? If you are unable to fully straighten it because it feels too tight at the back of the knee then you need to stretch those muscles. (see p. 47)

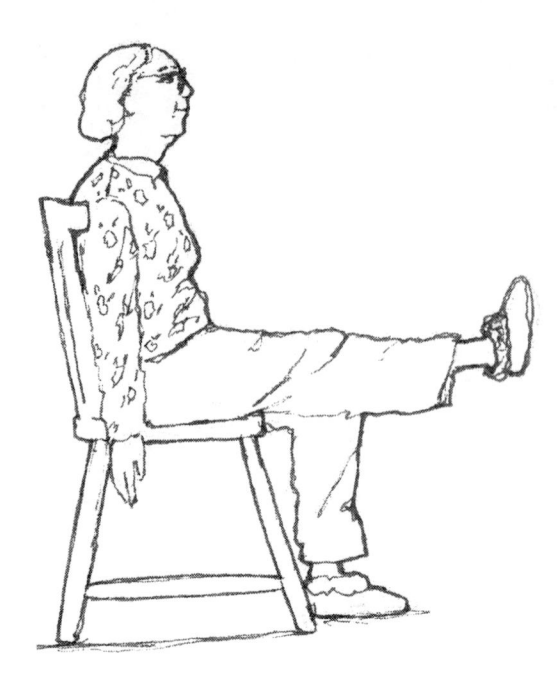

If you are unable to fully straighten it because the muscle just wont do that last bit, the leg feels too heavy or shaky, then it is important to strengthen those muscles and build up their stamina. Do this by repeating this movement as an exercise very regularly.

If your leg muscles feel tired this may be a sign that they are not strong enough for what you are asking them to do. You will really notice the difference if you take the trouble to strengthen them. You can do this by gradually increasing the distance you walk, by going up and downstairs, by doing sets of strengthening exercises. It may take some persistence – but well worth the effort.

The Kneecap/ Patella. A common problem is sharp pain at the front of the knee and a grating feeling on movement. This often occurs in teenage years but can develop at any age. It is usually caused by the kneecap being slightly tilted or pulled to the side. It then is not running smoothly in its groove and catches on the underlying bone. It is necessary to regain the correct balance between the muscles which control the kneecap, by stretching one side and strengthening the other. A physio will show you how. Sometimes it helps to use tape to hold the kneecap in the correct position for a while until the muscles adjust.

Hips

The hip is a wonderfully stable joint. You just have to look at the way it's designed - a large ball fitting into a deep socket. And then good strong muscles all around it. Of course it has to take our weight whether we are lying, sitting, standing or walking on it. It's hard to imagine anything could go wrong with it, but we all know of someone who has had to have it replaced. This is usually a very successful operation but why is it necessary?

- Some people have a hereditary or congenital problem where the ball is flatter or the socket not so deep. This makes it less stable.

- Some people fall and break the bone just below the ball. This often does not heal well, especially in older people, so it is better to replace the ball.

- If the compressive forces through the joint are greater than normal the joint surfaces are more likely to wear e.g. by being overweight, or having tight, tense muscles that pull the bones too closely together.

- People who walk with a marked sway will put a shearing force through hips and knees and this may damage the protective cartilage. This may be due to muscle weakness on the outer side of the hip. It can also irritate the bursa (a protective pad) on the side of the hip.

Pain originating in the hip joint will be felt deep in the groin or buttock.

If we sit for long periods, with the hips in a bent position, the joint stiffens and the muscles at the front of the hips tend to shorten. Then when we get up and walk it is difficult to take a good stride as this pulls against the short muscle. We feel stiff and may have to over-arch the back to compensate.

Of course if we don't use the muscles they will become weaker and then there is less protection and support around the joint.

People who walk with their feet turned out a lot place the hips in an incorrect position and the balance between the muscles is upset.

The answer to these problems is to walk regularly, with the feet pointing forwards, and avoiding a sway. Imagine you are balancing something on your head. Think tall.

- If you have to sit for long, try to get into the habit of stretching the front of the hip when you stand up.
- If you are already stiff, lie on your tummy and relax there for 10 minutes every day. This will gradually stretch you out

again and you will find that standing straight and walking become easier.
- If you already have painful hips keep them as flexible as possible, by moving them around in all directions and gently nudging the end of their range. Keep relaxed as you do this. They may feel especially stiff first thing in the morning so move them around before you get out of bed. The more flexible you can keep them the less likely they are to be painful.
- It often eases the hip to apply traction to the joint in order to create some space: stand sideways on a step, let the painful leg dangle over the edge of the step – notice the feeling of stretch around the joint – and then gently swing the leg.
- Keep the muscles strong. Can you stand on one leg, keeping your body directly over your leg? Can you go upstairs without having to pull up on the bannister?

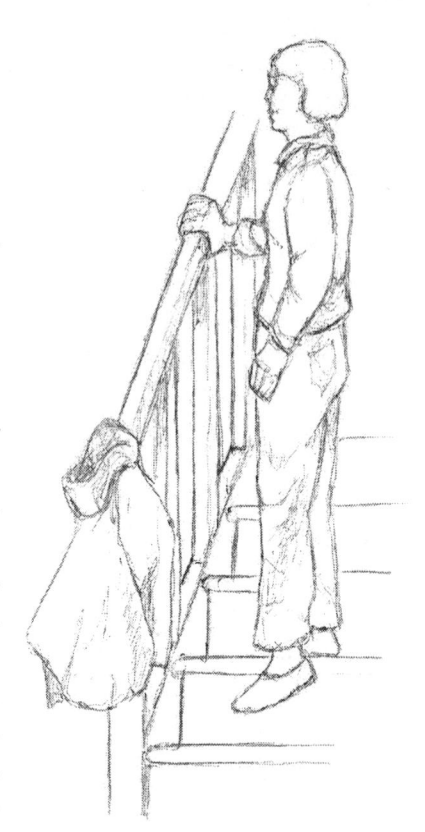

If these are difficult, practice doing them, until they become easy.

Hands to Shoulders

Hands

Some of the earliest cave paintings are of hands. Is this because even then humans appreciated what an advantage these extra-ordinarily skilful tools gave us over the other animals?

There are so many nerves going to the hands providing very quick and

An Easy Guide to Maintaining a Comfortable (and good looking) Body

efficient communication between the brain and the hands. And so we are able to do remarkable things, such as tying a knot, manipulating a fine tool, playing an instrument, even with our eyes closed. Our sense of touch, especially if we are blind, is wonderfully discriminating.

Hands can also be strong enough to wield a hammer or open a jar or cling to a rock-face.

Like the feet there are 28 bones, which all need to be able to move on each other, in order to provide the variety of skills we require.

There are many small muscles that allow us to move our fingers in many different ways. But the star of the hand is the thumb and the way it can move away from the rest of the hand, swing right round and across the palm. This gives us the ability to grip something firmly and also gives us the fine control of bringing thumb and index finger together. It is this movement which gives us such an advantage.

Hands also express our personality. Most people use their hands to gesticulate, to bring emphasis to what they are saying, and indeed create a whole method of communication if we are unable to speak.

Imagine having no hands. What a terrible disability that would be. So take care of them. Mostly they look after themselves because what they like is movement and that is what we are doing with our daily activities. Just don't let them stiffen or weaken through lack of use.

If you regularly sit for several hours, (perhaps watching TV), with your hands motionless on your lap, they are likely to stiffen, become a bit sluggish, and over time perhaps lose some of their skill. So do remember to move them every now and then; perhaps do some craft-work.

- Make sure you maintain a good span by stretching the fingers apart, and especially the thumb, as wide as you can.
- When you grip or hold something make sure the thumb forms a wide circle with the other fingers. If it is too close to the index finger the joint at the base of the thumb will be twisted and strained, especially with much repetition. (I notice that texting often twists the thumb like this. I wonder what the long term results will be.)

Enjoy the variety of activities these skilful tools of ours can do.

Some people develop arthritis in the fingers. The joints need lubricating and will feel better if you move them, gently pull on them, massage them. They often like a soak in warm water too. Prevent them stiffening by regular stretching

Pins and Needles in the hand

A feeling of pins and needles suggests there is an irritation of the nerves that supply that area. True numbness i.e. you can't feel that place if you touch it, indicates pressure on the nerve. The difficulty is to locate this irritation or pressure. In the hand it could be coming from the neck, upper back, shoulder, elbow, or wrist. This may be identified by which fingers are affected. It is always sensible to create the feeling of having a long neck, in order to make sufficient space for nerves which come from there. (see p. 35)

<u>**Carpal Tunnel Syndrome:**</u> one of the main nerves to the fingers, the median nerve, travels through a tunnel formed by some of the carpal bones in the hand and a fibrous band which holds that nerve and the tendons in place. If this tunnel is constricted for any reason there will be pressure on the nerve, irritating it, and pins and needles will be felt in the thumb, index, middle and ring fingers. This can be an intense tingling and often disturbs sleep. One cause may be sleeping with the wrist curled forwards, perhaps tucked under a cheek, as this position can compress the carpal tunnel. If pressure continues numbness and weakness can develop. Try to avoid this position by straightening your wrist; by changing that habit. Sometimes it helps to wear a wrist splint at night. If this does not help and the problem continues an injection or surgery may be necessary.

Pregnant women sometimes develop carpal tunnel syndrome, due to retaining extra fluid. It should settle soon after the birth.

The Wrist.

What happens when we trip or slip and fall? We put out our hand – usually the dominant hand – and land heavily on it. Often this results in a break of one or both bones, the Radius and Ulna, near to the wrist. Then, inconveniently we are in plaster for 4-6 weeks. Usually we can't write, do up buttons and all the other things we constantly need our hand for. And then, at last, the plaster is taken off. Oh no! - the wrist and thumb are painful and weak and the skin horribly flaky.

Advice: while in plaster don't be afraid to move the shoulder, elbow and fingers. In fact movement will improve the circulation – and therefore the healing, - and maintain the mobility of the joints and some strength in the muscles.

When the plaster is removed soak the hand in warm water, and then massage in plenty of oil or hand cream. Then start regaining the movement. It will feel very stiff and painful at first because it has been still for several weeks and no joint likes that. Exercise wrist and fingers and thumb. Start using it for everyday activities. Don't be fearful – the plaster would not have been removed if the bones were not united. It is important to regain FULL mobility within a few weeks otherwise it will probably always be restricted. So keep working away at it.

Sometimes it isn't possible to align the bones perfectly. You may notice a bump on the side of your wrist and may not be able to regain 100% movement – but work on restoring as much as possible.

It will of course feel weak; muscles weaken when not used. Don't expect it to be able to lift weights at first. But keep using it and gradually you will regain that strength.

<u>Repetitive Strain Injury – Upper limb work related disorders</u>
Working at a computer or any repetitive hand activities puts a great demand on the tendons around the wrist. They therefore need a good blood supply to give them the extra energy. Tendons do not naturally have a good blood supply but their attached muscles do – unless the blood flow is reduced. That can happen if we hold tension in our shoulder and forearm muscles, thereby squeezing the blood vessels, and unfortunately that is quite a common problem for those working at a computer or a factory bench..
This can lead to painful, stiff, weak hands and sometimes changes in sensation.

- Make sure you have a good posture. (see p. 38)
- Keep checking that your shoulders are relaxed. If, when you 'let them go' you notice that they drop down this will tell you that you have been holding tension there; a good reason to keep checking and then, hopefully, you will break the habit.
- Try to get in the habit of wriggling your shoulders frequently.

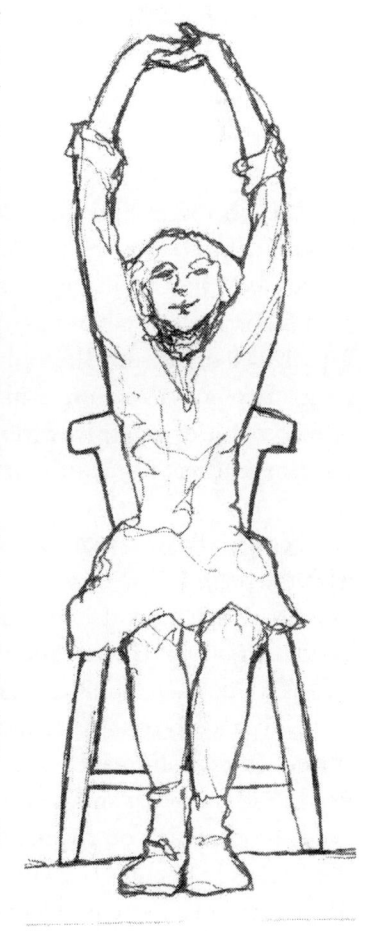

- Regularly get up and walk around.
- Every half hour stretch your hands and shoulders e.g. interlock your fingers, turn your palms down and then forwards, straighten your elbows, stretch your arms above your head. Hold there for 10 seconds. This becomes easier with repetition.
- Stretch your forearm muscles. (see p. 51)

If you know that you wont remember to do this half-hourly then take an oven-timer to work and set the bell to ring – that might make your colleagues interested and they could do it too! Or arrange some sign to flash up on your computer – but please don't ignore it. Quite quickly this will become a habit and you won't need the timer any more.

Remember that prevention is much better than cure. Once you have the problem it can be difficult to resolve. You may well have to take time off work, see a specialist, wear a splint etc.

Elbows

The most vital elbow movement is to bring the hand to the mouth – a smooth combination of bending and rotating. If you break a bone near to the elbow it is critical to recover that movement. You wouldn't want to starve! Fortunately elbows are pretty workmanlike joints and keep going happily all our lives. The only common complaint is Tennis elbow or sometimes Golfer's elbow. Usually these occur for other reasons than sport, often because of repetitive actions that inflame and create scar-tissue in the forearm tendons which originate at the elbow.

Tennis elbow – pain and tenderness on the thumb side of the elbow with the palm facing forwards - is the most frequent because those are the muscles which extend / cock-up the wrist. This occurs whenever we grip or hold anything. If the tendon is inflamed it hurts when we do this action and as we do this a lot it can be very disabling.

Golfer's elbow – pain and tenderness on the little finger side of the elbow – is less common because it is due to a problem in the muscles which flex / bend our wrist and we don't use those so much. But there are certain occupations which do require repetitive wrist flexion and that can irritate the tendon.

Advice for both these problems:

- Avoid repetitive, painful movements.
- Unless the pain is acute – in which case an ice pack may help – gently and regularly stretch the tight (probably scarred) muscle. Warmth may help before or while you are stretching.
- If you play a raquet sport remember to stretch the forearm muscles after the game. It may help to use a raquet with a wider handle if you feel any discomfort.
- A tennis elbow band may help but usually it is no good simply wrapping it round your forearm. It needs to alter the angle of pull of the muscle and that entails drawing the muscle over to one side. Then fasten the band. If gripping is then comfortable you know you have positioned it correctly.

Like all tendon problems they can take a long time to resolve. A physio may be able to help you further.

Shoulders

Our shoulders do a remarkable job. They provide the greatest flexibility in the body but also need to be strong. We use them to reach, throw, push and pull, carry, and co-ordinate all the movements of the arms. We expect them to be able to twist into extraordinary positions – doing the back of our hair, tucking in a shirt, turning off the bedside light. We expect them to be able to keep going for a hundred years and can become quite upset if they complain. It pays to understand how they work and give them some attention.

A shoulder joint is made up of 3 bones: the shoulder-blade/scapula, the collar-bone/clavicle, and the upper arm/humerus. These bones have to work together with absolute precision. The joint itself needs to be unstable; otherwise it couldn't be so mobile. There needs to be space between the ball of the humerus and the socket of the scapula to permit such freedom of movement.

The stability comes from the supporting muscles.

The key to the system is the position of the shoulder-blades. These flat "wing" bones should be tucked back, lying against the rib-cage, held in that position by the muscles attached to them.

Try pulling your shoulder-blades together, back and down, and be aware of those muscles. Then let them relax but not so much that the shoulders droop forwards. This should be our habitual position, whether we are sitting, standing, walking, lifting or carrying. This position places the three bones, and therefore the shoulder joint, in the correct position to allow the joint to move smoothly and the muscles to work efficiently.

When we reach above shoulder level the blade slides around the ribs causing the joint to point upwards and then the muscles can work in the same way but at a higher level. Good co-ordination between muscles is required for this movement to occur smoothly.

The shoulders and neck will work more comfortably if the shoulders are level and relaxed down. Have a look at people carrying shoulder bags. Notice how they are inclined to hunch the shoulder the bag is on. The bit of tension required for this can easily become a habit and continue at all times. Far better to use a backpack or a bag with a strap that goes across the chest. Interestingly if you tension and hunch one shoulder this will be balanced by tension in the opposite low back muscles. Shoulder and back problems often go together – and to cure one you may have to cure both!

The muscles provide strength and control. There is a group of muscles which wrap around the shoulder joint, holding it in position and co-ordinating all movements - the Rotator Cuff muscles. They need to be able to perform those most complex of movements – rotating or twisting the arm – as well as holding the arm in its optimum position.

Once the joint is in a correct position, and the Rotator Cuff muscles controlling that, then the action muscles can perform with confidence.

E.g.: when pushing up from a chair or walking using a stick we should use the large muscles which run from the shoulders down the back combined with those down the back of our arms. This will keep our shoulders down and in the correct, strong position. If instead the pressure pushes our shoulders upwards we subject them to huge forces in a weakened position. With repetition they are likely to be damaged.

Lifting and carrying – a group of muscles work together to spread the load, especially if we share it between both arms. This system works well, as long as we don't try to lift or carry a weight that is too great for us, and as long as our shoulder- blades are in that backward and downward position. If the shoulders are rounded forwards, however, this places excessive strain on the small muscles, ligaments and joints around the shoulder. Tendons are likely to be pinched between the bones causing swelling, inflammation and scarring. It is even possible, when we are older, for the tendon to frey and tear. Developing the habit of a good posture can prevent all this.

People who sit a lot – in their armchair, at a computer, at a workbench, driving, - often slump, causing the shoulders to round forwards. This can become a habit and feel correct. The muscles at the back can become over-

An Easy Guide to Maintaining a Comfortable (and good looking) Body

stretched and weak; the muscles at the front can become shortened and tight. You have lost the correct position and your shoulders are vulnerable. Be aware and correct this. You have been warned! Do not let your shoulders droop forwards, especially when they are having to work hard. You may get away with it for some time and then suddenly some small, twisting movement or an unexpected pull will be the final straw.

> The Acromio-Clavicular joint. This is the little joint between the collar-bone and the shoulder-blade and it may become damaged or worn if too much pressure goes onto it. You wouldn't think that long-distance lorry driving would pressurise it but in fact if you sit with your arms stretched in front of you, hands in the ten-to-two position, for hundreds of miles every day, it certainly can begin to give trouble and the pain can be very sharp. I have seen many drivers with this problem, though usually they can't find time to attend regularly for treatment. Fortunately advice alone often helps. Yet again the tip is to draw those shoulder-blades back so that the chest widens and there is no weight going through the joints. And also to wriggle the shoulders frequently.

Check list:
- ▶ Is your head balanced above your body?
- ▶ Are your shoulder-blades positioned back and down?
- ▶ Are your shoulders relaxed?
- ▶ Are your shoulders level? You may need to check this in a mirror.
- ▶ Have you moved your shoulders around during the last half-hour?
- ▶ Can you stretch your arms above your head? Can you stretch them backwards? If not work towards being able to do so.

If your shoulder is painful and none of this helps, you should see your GP or Physio.

Frozen shoulder / Capsulitis – this is a common problem affecting people between the ages of 40 and 60. The cause at present is uncertain. The tissue surrounding the joint – the capsule – becomes inflamed and very painful. This is often worse at night. The shoulder then becomes very stiff, blocking movement in all directions. Unfortunately the problem lasts for 18 months to two years but the pain does lessen and eventually the stiffness goes too.

- Find out what helps to reduce the pain. Your doctor will advise you about medication.
- You may also find that ice-packs help to reduce the inflammation.
- You may find that warmth helps by relaxing the muscles.
- Finding a comfortable position at night can be difficult. Resting the arm on a pillow may help.
- Move the arm about gently and regularly, keeping as much movement as possible, but don't force through pain.
- Once pain has settled start exercising and stretching more vigorously in order to regain all the movements.
- Keep cheerful; it will go away!

The Spine

The spine is the chain that links everything together. It is complex and fascinating, - and can be troublesome. It demands a whole book to itself and indeed there are many books and thousands of articles about this area of the body. I will try not to get too carried away!

It is made up of good strong blocks of bone - the vertebrae, with shock-absorbing cushions - the discs, joining them together. These are larger at the bottom of the spine, where they have to take more weight, and get smaller further up, with the smallest vertebrae situated in the neck. The side joints (facet joints) between each vertebra are very small, only allowing quite small movement at each one, but as there are 24 vertebrae this adds up to plenty of movement for all our activities.

There are short muscles and ligaments between each vertebra holding them in place and making necessary adjustments as we move.

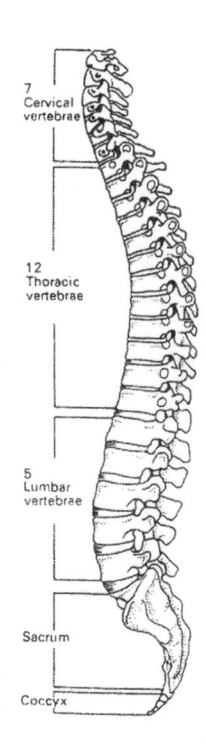

There are longer muscles and other connective tissue, acting like guy ropes, which assist keeping the spine in whatever position we are in but also linking the spine with the limbs. These "guy ropes" have to be elastic to cope with the constant changes, but like guy ropes on a tent they need to be the right length to work effectively.

All the nerves which send messages to and from the brain pass through a channel created by the shape of the vertebrae. At each level nerves emerge from this spinal cord so instructions can be sent to specific muscles. A constant stream of information from those muscles, and the skin, joints etc. go along nerves to the brain in order to maintain and alter the position of the body with ease.

There is a vast network of blood vessels to cope with the demands for oxygen and nutrition and the removal of waste products at this busy part of the body.

The Neck / Cervical Spine

- A head is very heavy – 10 to 15 pounds (5-7 kilos). Work out how many bags of sugar that is! If it is balanced over the rest of our body there isn't much strain but if it is in front of that plumb-line there will be a big pull on the muscles and a shearing force on those very small joints and discs. Feel for your breastbone. Is your chin directly above that? That is where it should be, and balancing there comfortably. If this is not easy you may have to stretch the base of your neck, (see p. 50) and keep reminding yourself of the correct position, until it does become easy, comfortable and your new habit.

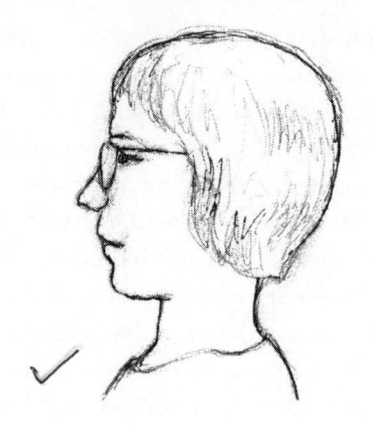

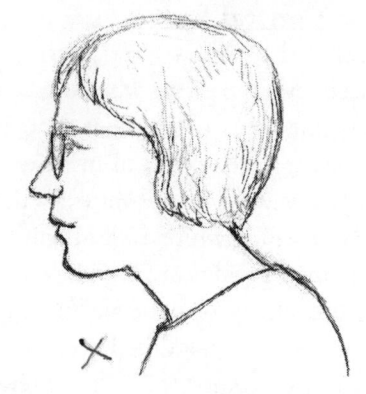

> Headaches and Dizziness. The nerves from the upper part of the neck supply the head and face, so headaches and dizziness may be due to a neck problem, though there are many causes. One poor man had been investigated for months for his severe and persistent headaches. When nothing could be found on brain scans etc., he was finally sent to physiotherapy. After two treatments on the stiff, tender section of his neck his headaches ceased and he could sleep without problems. A few more treatments were required, largely to retrain his posture.

The nerves from the lower part of the neck supply the shoulder and arm. Therefore symptoms of pain, pins and needles, numbness can be felt in those areas. If you have any of those symptoms remember to make your neck as long as possible to make space for those nerves.

Maintain full mobility, moving the head in all directions. If a particular position makes you dizzy avoid it and ask advice.

Do you spend a lot of time on the telephone? Notice if you hold it in place by tilting your head and hunching your shoulder. That position could easily pinch a nerve.

Notice when you are driving or on the computer whether your chin tends to poke forwards. This position is also likely to create problems, especially if held for a long time and becomes habitual.

<u>Cervical Spondylosis</u> is a common diagnosis for those with neck pain. That sounds pretty serious and often makes people anxious. I have seen several patients who come with extremely stiff necks because they have assumed this means that their bones are 'fusing' or perhaps 'crumbling' and they are fearful of moving too much. In fact it means that there are signs of wear in the spine, which happens to us all, as we age – like my hair turning white. Like all joints they like the pressure taken off them - by having a good posture and by avoiding tension in the muscles around them - and plenty of natural, lubricating movement. The crackling sounds in the neck are magnified because the joints are so close to our ears. If I hear 'crackles' I know that I have tensed up and my posture is incorrect. They cease when I relax and adjust my posture. When lying use a soft pillow which tucks into and supports your neck. A feather pillow usually works well – unless you are allergic to them.

Thoracic Spine

The more flexible this part of the spine is the easier it is for the neck and shoulders to move. The better the posture here the better the position of the neck and head. This is also the part of the spine that the ribs are attached to. It is important to keep all those little rib joints moving well as of course it is vital that we are able to breathe easily. How can we do that? Well, by taking a few really deep breaths every now and then, while sitting or standing in a good posture.

- It is also a good idea to stretch our arms up towards the ceiling, as that also stretches the muscles between the ribs. Try this and feel the stretch through the rib cage.
- Sit and swivel – so one shoulder moves backwards and the other forwards. This movement will not only maintain good mobility but also benefit the many nerves and blood vessels in this region. Those nerves and blood vessels supply a large area of the body, so symptoms can be widespread – down the arms, around the rib-cage, into the abdomen; almost anywhere in fact as some of these nerves supply blood vessels and the blood vessels supply nerves. Remember to position the shoulder-blades correctly as this helps to maintain a good position in this part of the spine. If we allow ourselves to slump the lungs and stomach will be squashed and wont function as well, - and we look older.

Lumbar Spine

It is said that 80% of the population in the western world will have back pain at some time in their life. Is this something to do with our lifestyle, as it is far less of a problem in other cultures?
If you have seen films of people walking in Africa or Asia you can see how well they hold themselves – tall, straight and often balancing something on their heads, which they wouldn't be able to do if they swayed from side to side or stooped.
Often they do not have chairs and so may squat – an excellent position for the back – or sit on the ground with legs straight out in front, demonstrating good flexibility of muscles and nerves.

Most people cannot afford a car so they walk or cycle long distances – keeping themselves very fit.

Most people are not over-weight, so their bodies are not having to continuously carry more than they should.

I spent some years working in Africa and the only time I treated a person with back pain was someone who had adopted a western lifestyle – sitting at a desk, driving a car, putting on some weight. Apart that is from those patients with TB (tuberculosis) spine, which fortunately for us in the western world is now uncommon, or a fractured spine.

The major causes of back problems are:
- Poor posture
- Poor flexibility
- Poor muscle control and fitness
- Joints, discs, muscles under strain from carrying too much weight, whether our own or an outside force.
- Poor circulation – this may be due to heavy smoking or holding tension in the back muscles.
- Some people do seem to inherit a back problem; all the more reason to learn how to keep it functioning well.

When you are in pain you want a diagnosis. It does make it easier then to understand what is happening and how to cope with it. This isn't always easy with the spine as there are so many structures involved and often it is a combination of these.

Intervertebral Disc – a 'slipped disc' is a frequent diagnosis. I would be very anxious if I knew my disc had slipped out of place but fortunately this is impossible. The fibrous outer casing of the disc is attached firmly to the adjacent vertebrae. However if a split occurs in this casing some of the inner jelly-like substance can squeeze through and irritate or press on neighbouring nerves. This is more likely to occur if we sit slumped, or put a sudden force onto the spine, or repetitively bend and twist.

By middle-age the 'jelly' is drying out so unable to squeeze through. This does mean that the disc becomes thinner so there is a little less space between the small facet joints. With the extra compression of excess weight, or poor posture, or sudden strains, these joints may be damaged – especially if the protective muscles are not functioning well.

Chronic back pain: - Ongoing and recurrent back pain. Vast sums of money are spent on treatments of various kinds and those suffering have huge expectations of finding a cure, from surgery, injections, manipulations etc., and indeed sometimes these work – for a while. But the most effective long-

An Easy Guide to Maintaining a Comfortable (and good looking) Body

term treatment is what you do yourself, so that **you** are in control. It often helps to have someone who has an expertise in spinal problems to assess your back – and then advise you what it is necessary for you to do to improve the situation.

Look at the list above of common causes, look at yourself critically, and take control.

- Think tall, whether sitting or standing or walking. Persist with this until it becomes your natural habit and you no longer have to think about it. (see p. 34/35)
- Keep active, move around, change position, 'wriggle', especially if you have been still for a while. Try those gentle exercises described in the section on Lubrication. Prolonged resting will make your back worse.
- Stretch anything that appears to be stiff or tight. (see p. 48 and picture on p. 62)
- Learn how to let go of any tension, (see p. 41) and how to move easily and gracefully.
- Learn how to lift safely. (see p. 37) Strong muscles will protect your spine.
- Make sure your bed gives you good, comfortable support.
- If your stomach protrudes forwards this will pull mightily on the spine. In addition the supporting stomach muscles will become over-stretched, lax and weak. It is really worthwhile strengthening those muscles and adjusting your posture , to prevent chronic back pain.

Be prepared for it to take a little time for these suggestions to become habitual and effective but it is so worthwhile. You can save yourself years of discomfort.

Sitting to standing

It can often be quite painful moving from sitting to standing – especially if the seat is low or soft. Once your body knows it is going to be painful it tightens in anticipation. It is easier if you sit on a higher chair, but it also helps to use your strong hips instead of your back. The hip joint is positioned deep in the groin area. Move forward on the chair, bend from the hips until you can feel the weight going through your feet, thrust down through your feet and straighten your knees – and you are standing. Many people then find that their back didn't take the strain, and therefore didn't hurt

Acute Back pain: - what a nightmare! Your back is twingeing, you can't move or find a comfortable position, your life has ground to a halt. It is so painful you start imagining all sorts of awful reasons for it. And often all you did was pick up something really light. Or perhaps you woke up with it. Or perhaps you slipped on a wet rock and landed flat on your back, as I did when walking in the mountains. In my case I had to keep walking as the nearest hut to stay in was 3 hours away. Very painful it was too; my husband found me a stick and on we went. And gradually the pain lessened until 3 hours later it was only an ache – and the next morning it had gone. What this story shows is how important it is to move, even if it is the last thing you feel like doing. I have also frequently seen people who have been told to 'lie down until it gets better.' This is a BAD idea. It will indeed eventually improve but probably more slowly than if they had not gone to bed, and the scenario is set for future back problems.

What should one do? Don't panic! Yes, it is painful but it is almost certainly not serious and it will settle down.

Your muscles will have gone into spasm and are jamming the little joints together.

- Find your most comfortable position, take a painkiller or anti-inflammatory if you find they help, and try hard to relax those muscles. An ice-pack or warmth may help. Find out which helps you the most.
- Start to move very gently; small movements which don't hurt. Deep breathing might be one of those movements and will also help you to relax. Always do these movements before getting out of bed.
- If you are lying flat and sit straight up your back will hate it. There will be much less strain if you bend your knees; roll onto your side with knees, hips, shoulders and head all rolling together; take your lower legs over the side of the bed; then sit up, keeping your back straight.
- Then begin to walk about. It will be uncomfortable at first but will gradually get easier. Certainly faster than if you don't move.

You may have to modify your activities for a day or two – not easy I know when, for example, you have a young family to look after. You may have to ask for help. At first you may find that it is a real struggle to get dressed in the morning – you are fighting the tightness and the fear of hurting yourself - and so the day starts badly. My advice is to leave dressing until you have had breakfast, giving your body time to free itself. Gradually increase the amount you are doing.

Once it has settled make sure you regain full flexibility and strength.

'Sciatica' : if you are getting shooting pain and/ or pins and needles down your leg, one of the nerves is being irritated. This may be because the channel through which the nerve passes out from the spinal cord has become too small for comfort. There are various reasons for this but it is worth trying to make the channel wider by thinking tall - lifting your upper body up so that it is not compressing your lower spine, and relaxing your back muscles so your tail hangs down, creating some space between the joints. Look at the advice for acute back pain, above.
When sleeping it may be more comfortable to lie on the opposite side to the pain and tuck a small pillow under your waist.

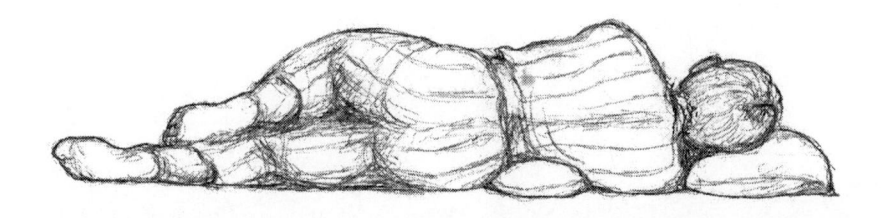

When lying in this position I find that gently rocking the top leg forwards and back, just an inch or so and without lifting it, works well. Don't stop moving about as this will not help, but go a bit more gently than usual.

It is quite common to have had several episodes of back pain over some years and then suddenly develop sciatica. Once the nerve is irritated it can take several weeks for it to settle. If it doesn't improve you need further help, so discuss this with your doctor or therapist. See him/her urgently if you have symptoms of weakness or numbness in both legs or difficulty passing urine.

About 2% of people with sciatica will need a scan with a view to surgery or injection.

Sacro-Iliac joint:

This is the very solid joint between the sacrum/tail bone and the pelvis. It is a frequent site for discomfort but it is rarely the cause of that discomfort. Usually pain is referred there from the low back. The only time it is likely to cause trouble is during pregnancy. This is because the immensely strong ligaments which unite the two bones slacken to permit the pelvis to widen and to allow for the birth. Those ligaments will firm up again after the birth. It sometimes helps, during pregnancy, to wear a sacro-iliac belt. It certainly helps to be aware of the correct posture to limit drag on that area. You will be given advice in your ante-natal classes.

The joint can be irritated if it is mis-aligned. The most likely cause for this is falling heavily onto it. I have seen a few keen horse-riders with this problem! The joint may then need to be re-aligned by a physio or osteopath.

A marked difference in leg length can affect the Sacro-Iliac joint and the spine. An insole to adjust that may then help.

Chapter 3.
Physical Skills for Easy Living.

The best way to maintain a comfortable body is to have the right habits of posture, movement and activity. Then you won't need to give it much thought. Perhaps you already have those habits - but it may be worth checking. In this chapter I will discuss some of the necessary body skills. **How to develop a new habit:** Firstly decide that it makes good sense to do so. Then think about it and practice it frequently; use every opportunity, every day. It may help to ask family and friends to remind you. Find reminder triggers: notes, messages, alarm bells, whatever works for you. The change may take 2 – 3 weeks but should become easier all the time. Once established you don't have to worry anymore - just the occasional check – and you will save yourself so much time and discomfort.

<u>Posture</u>

When we meet someone for the first time we instantly form an impression of them. If they are smiling and welcoming we warm to them. If their brow is furrowed and their shoulders hunched we guess they are anxious and stressed. If they are stooped we think they are old – perhaps older than they actually are. Many people say that they have always been like that; that their parents were always telling them to stand up straight. Perhaps they visually picked up the habit from the people around them; perhaps they were growing faster than their friends and didn't want to be different; perhaps they sat in front of the TV or computer for long hours. Perhaps you still do…

Standing and walking - Stooping is not kind to the body. It puts far more strain on the neck, shoulders and back than when you are upright. It shortens some muscles and weakens others so that your "guy ropes" are unbalanced. It also compresses your inner organs and may lead to stomach or breathing problems.

The way you sit, stand and move will have become a habit and so will feel "right". It may be - but it may not. Look at yourself critically in a long mirror. Are you straight? Can you imagine a plumb-line down through your body?

If your feet roll in this will twist your knees and hips at every step. If your head bends down or pokes forward this will strain your neck, shoulders and upper back. It is not worth it; it is likely to cause wear of the cartilage and joints, pinching of tendons, - and pain.

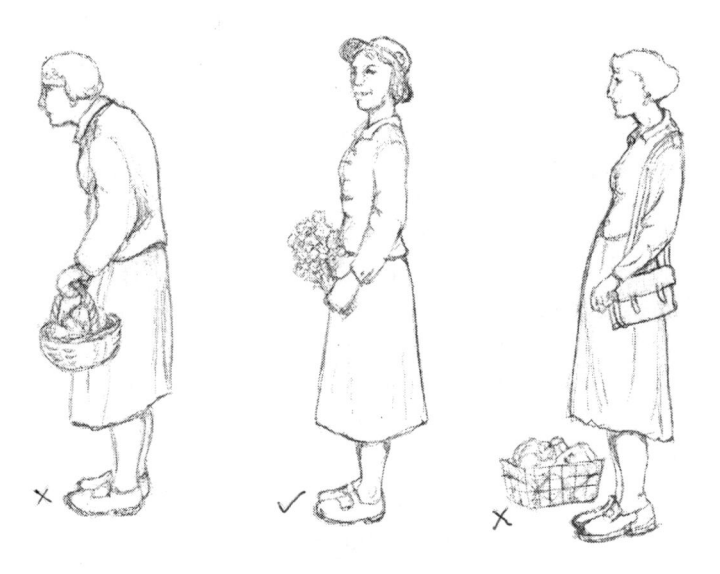

Simply by developing the habit of a correct posture you can prevent or reduce all kinds of problems. It is well worth the effort.

Check list in standing:
- Equal weight on heels and the balls of your feet
- Instep slightly raised

- Knees soft, not pushed back.
- Your pelvis is a bowl which contains the inner organs. If it is tilted forwards those organs will tend to protrude and drag on your spine. In order to position the pelvis correctly feel that your tail-bone is hanging down and your navel drawn back,.
- A long waistline, i.e. a good space between your pelvis and rib-cage, so that the spinal joints and discs, and the nerves, are not being compressed.
- Back muscles relaxed. It is the deep muscles that hold the vertebrae in place, not the ones you can feel under the skin.
- Shoulder blades tucked back; minimum tension to hold them in place.
- Shoulders down and relaxed.
- Head floating up, creating a long neck; plenty of space for those nerves and blood vessels, but no tension.

Now can you walk around while maintaining that feeling of being tall? All the time?

Something to do while waiting at the check-out, or at a bus stop – or anywhere.

Imagine that you have a horse's tail, hanging straight down, and that your head is a balloon filled with helium, so it feels it is floating up!

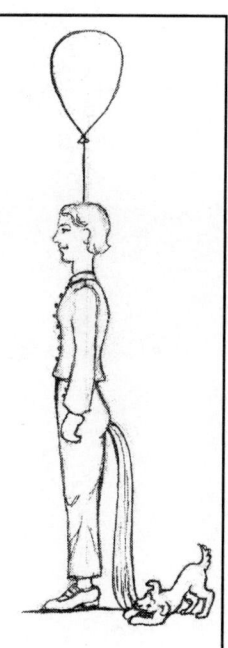

This posture will make you look younger, feel better (and more elegant!) and you will be far less likely to suffer from recurrent back, neck or shoulder pain. You will also naturally tone up the supporting muscles that you need. Notice that if you place your fingers on your tummy muscles while walking like this you can feel them working. Easier than sit-ups!

If you use a walking aid continue to think tall. Avoid leaning forward over it, which is all too easy to do, or you will quickly become stooped.

Carrying - Notice the position of other people's shoulders and spine when they are carrying a heavy bag in one hand or on one shoulder. Do you carry one? Could you use a back pack or distribute the weight between two bags? Or use wheels?

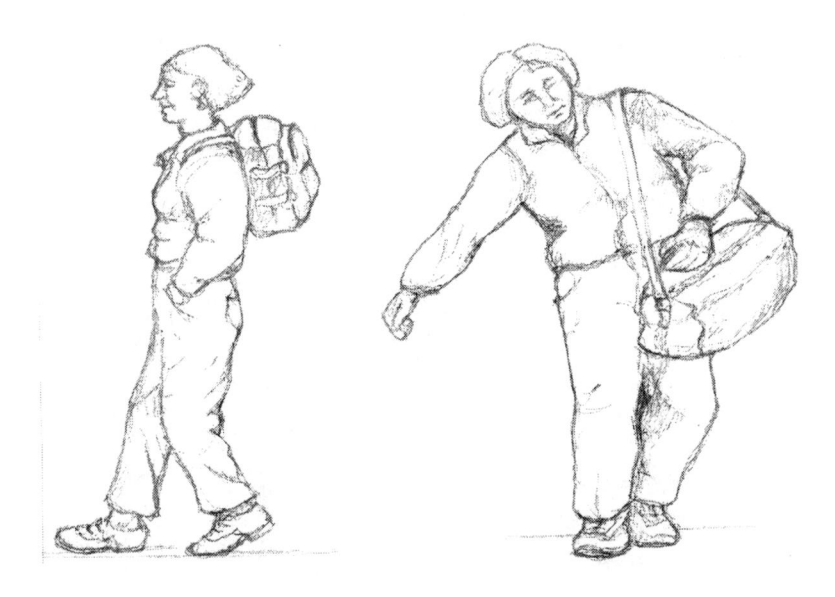

An Easy Guide to Maintaining a Comfortable (and good looking) Body

> **Lifting**
> - Keep your hips lower than your back, have your feet apart and use strong leg muscles to do the work – not your back.
> - Pull your tummy in. This helps to support your back.
> - Set your shoulder-blades back and down.
> - Keep the load close to you. Lifting a weight on an outstretched arm creates far more strain than lifting it with a bent elbow close to your body.
> - Do not twist while lifting. If you point one foot in the direction you are coming from and the other in the direction you are lifting to, you will pivot on your strong hips rather than twist your more vulnerable back.
> - Ask for help if the object is awkward or too heavy for you.

Sitting - One of the causes of poor posture is poor furniture – sofas and armchairs that encourage us to slump because they are too soft, too low, too long in the leg for us. And we may sit like this for hours because we are absorbed in some fascinating TV programme. Difficult to get up? Stiff? Research has shown that more pressure goes onto the spinal discs in sitting, especially slumped sitting, than in any other position, so make sure that you have support for your low back which keeps it in a slightly arched position. The pressure on your spine will be even worse if it is twisted, so make sure that your TV or computer is straight in front of you, not to one side. It's worth thinking about - you can waste a lot of time dealing with a bad back or shoulder.

If you sit like this when you are a teenager and growing you are likely to over-stretch the ligaments and then will have poor support for the spine in the future. School furniture is often too low for the taller children and so they will slump over the table. The old-fashioned sloping desks placed the spine in a better position and I have seen some good designs for school furniture in Denmark.

It improves your position if you prop up the book you are reading so that you don't need to lean forward over it.

It feels good to sit sometimes in an upright chair with your arms looped over the back of the chair. This will place your shoulders and back in a better position, and you can relax because the chair is doing the work for you. Try it for a short time.

The problem may be that you spend many hours at a computer.

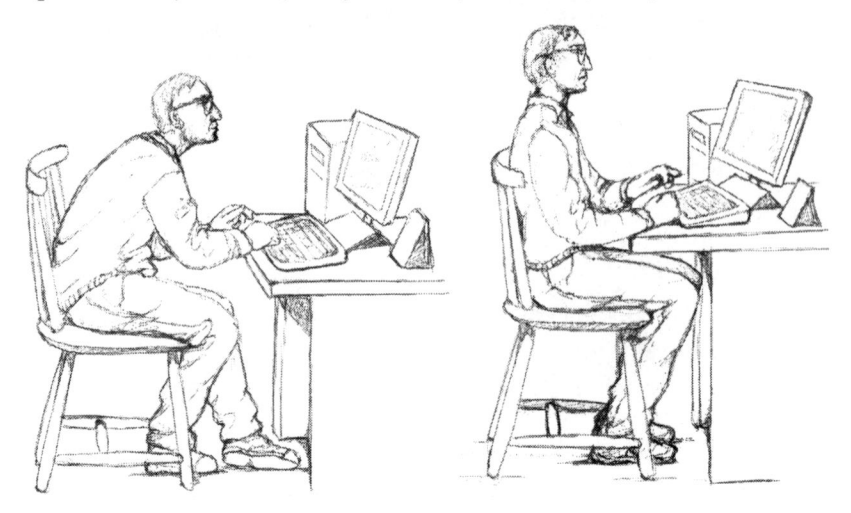

Checklist at the computer:
- ▶ Is the screen at eye level when you sit tall and is it straight in front of you – not to one side?
- ▶ Is the vision good or do you have to crane your neck forward?
- ▶ Can you get your legs right under the desk so your forearms are supported?
- ▶ Does your chair give you good support? Do you lean away from its back or sink into a slump? A kneeling-chair will usually place your back in a better position, but you still need to change position regularly or your knees may complain. Or try sitting on a wedge-shaped cushion so that your thighs are sloping down. Find out what suits you best; we are all different shapes and sizes.

Even if everything is perfect the body is not designed for this sort of work. Make sure that every half-hour you get up and walk around or at least have a good stretch. You may need a message on your screen or an alarm bell/oven timer to remind you at first.

Lying - What about lying in bed? It should be the time to relax and be comfortable. But if the bed is too soft your spine may be curved or twisted for hours. If the mattress is too hard it doesn't adapt to your curves, and that can be uncomfortable. Best to have a firm base and a good, thick mattress with some give in it. If you and your partner are very different weights it is often better to have two separate mattresses, and separate duvets, so you can move around without disturbing the other. Even when you are asleep nerves and blood vessels need space, so it's a good idea to check before going to sleep that you are not lying with your spine twisted, or your shoulders hunched, or your hands curled. Have a nice long stretch just before going to bed or when you first get in.

Too many pillows will push your spine into a rounded or twisted position. It is best to have one soft pillow which moulds into the shape of your neck and supports its normal curve.

Tension

In the forty plus years that I have been working as a physiotherapist I have treated thousands of people with all sorts of different conditions but pain has usually been an important factor. I have become convinced that a great deal of pain, especially when it has been continuing for a time, is due to tension. And very frequently those people have been quite unaware that they are holding tension - and anyway have no idea how to release it. If only we were more in tune with our bodies we could make the necessary small adjustments and save ourselves such a lot of discomfort. I have found this to be true as on the occasions when I have hurt myself I can quite quickly relieve the pain – by letting go tension and moving with ease. My body has been a useful laboratory!

If there has been some damage to part of the body the surrounding muscles will go into protective spasm. This prevents that part moving and may be useful at first. However if this muscle tension continues it will clamp the nearby joint together, preventing normal movement, reduce the lubrication of that joint, and slow blood flow which is so important for healing.

Good stress and bad stress

Bodies benefit from a certain amount of stress. As we put pressure onto our bones they respond by creating stronger bone. As we work our muscles, and other tissues, they get stronger.

When we are really involved in, even stressed by, some exciting activity or project it can make us feel truly alive.

In fact if consistently we take stress off our bones, i.e. by being very sedentary, by having a long period of time in bed, even by being underweight – they may lose some of their strength. If we don't use our muscles enough they will become weaker and less able to support our bodies. Limbs will feel "heavy"; activities will become more of an effort, balance can become shaky.

So a certain amount of stress is good. What our bodies do not like is a state of permanent tension, even at a low level. Our shoulder-girdle muscles are often called our "stress" muscles because they are a frequent site for tension. For some reason it is common to hold tension in those muscles, often hunching our shoulders, when we are stressed. Perhaps it was in readiness for throwing a spear when we were attacked by some great beast! They often tense when we are driving or working at a computer, or cold, or under pressure. Emotional stress can be even worse. This tension can very quickly become a habit, so we are not aware of it and it becomes permanent. The tightness in muscle will squeeze the blood vessels and slow blood flow. This means less oxygen and nutrition to both that muscle and to the tissues the blood vessels supply, so the discomfort can become more widespread. I am sure this frequently leads to repetitive strain injuries, work related disorders, tendon and nerve damage. Knots may occur in the muscles and these can become acutely tender. Tenderness may also occur due to the waste products in muscles not being adequately removed.
Just see how people love having their shoulders and neck massaged!
Tension is extremely fatiguing as we are working harder and longer than necessary.
As bones are pulled together by muscle tension there is a reduction in the space and freedom of movement in the joint. End range and accessory movements are reduced and that area stiffens up. Bones can be pulled into an incorrect position causing mal-alignment and incorrect posture.

Stress releases Adrenaline into the body. This is a useful chemical if we are in a fight or having to run from a situation. It stimulates the necessary muscles. It is not useful if it is continuous, as it also transfers blood away from some parts of the body to those "Fight/Flight" muscles. This can effect our digestion, our vision, even the way we think. It can make us more sensitive to pain too.

Tension → Pain → Tension

If this continues it is likely to lead to chronic pain.
This sounds awful – and it certainly can be – but we can prevent all of this happening.

Relaxation Techniques

This is such an important skill. If you feel you are tense and don't know how to relax do please learn how. Like any skill it takes some persistence but, like learning to ride a bicycle, if you persist you suddenly find you can. It does not mean being lazy. It results in you using your body efficiently. You don't have to lie down to be relaxed, though it may help when you are learning how. There are many different techniques; it is a matter of finding which one suits you.

Here are a few to try:

Deep breathing:

The one activity that we certainly all can do is breathing! But we can learn to use it to benefit the body even more, rather than simply to keep us alive. Breathing deeply will improve oxygen intake, so important for healthy tissues. It also stimulates Endorphins, those important chemicals which help us to be relaxed and counter-act too much Adrenaline. You may notice that when you breathe out deeply you can feel muscles relaxing.
Here are a few ways of using your breathing. You can do this in any position.
- As you breathe notice your chest rising and falling, your ribs expanding then relaxing in, your tummy rising and falling. Then deepen this breath - your tummy rises, then your ribs expand, then feel the breath going right up to your collar-bones. Hold it there for the count of two or three. Then let your chest fall, your ribs relax in, your tummy go in. Hold it there for the count of two or three. Do several deep breaths like this.
- Breathe in for the count of four, hold for four, breathe out for four, hold for four.
- Breathe in and think about your feet. Breathe out and let them soften. Breathe in and think about your knees. Breathe out and let them soften. Continue like this all through the body. Pay particular attention to any part you feel is holding tension or you know is uncomfortable.

Quick relaxation:

- One deep breath in; then as you sigh out make sure your shoulders relax down.

-'Stop and flop'. Be aware of your shoulders and let them relax down. If they do drop down you know you have been holding tension in them.

> **Something to do, for example, when stopped by traffic lights or jams.**
>
> Breathe in for the count of seven and out for the count of eleven. This takes a bit of practice but gets easier, and it is a great way to relax in a stressful situation.

Tense/Relax:

Often we are unaware we are holding tension. Sometimes it helps to deliberately tension muscles, hold for the count of five, and then let them relax – and notice the difference. Work through the whole body, starting at the feet and working up. Don't forget your face, all those little muscles around eyes, jaw and mouth, as this is a common place to hold tension. If you find you hold tension in a particular part of your body keep returning to that part.

Visualisation:

Let your imagination take over. Picture yourself in a favourite place, real or imaginary. Think about it in great detail – what can you see? What can you hear? What can you smell? What can you feel? Spend time enjoying it.

The more frequently you practice relaxing, the easier you will find it. This may lessen pain; it may help you to sleep; it certainly will take pressure off your body so it will be less fatigued.

If you are finding this difficult find someone who can teach you.

> A mother with two small children, working part-time to supplement her husband's income, and with an elderly father to look after who had recently been diagnosed with Alzheimer's, came to me complaining of neck and shoulder pain. This was making her already difficult life even more exhausting. It didn't help that she was also having problems with her teeth as she was grinding them at night and had to wear a brace. She was understandably very stressed. Once she realised the effects this tension was having on her body she worked hard on learning how to relax. This took a little time but she persisted as she quickly realised that the pain was much less when she was relaxed. In addition she stopped grinding her teeth once she stretched her jaw (page 50) before going to sleep, and so could abandon the brace. She still had a stressful life but without the additional problems.

Stretching

Why Stretch

Muscles need to be a certain length, to balance each other, and this allows us to move with ease. Because they are elastic their length changes as we use them: they shorten as we work them and lengthen as we relax. In order to do a movement the necessary muscles will contract and shorten and the opposing muscles, on the other side of the joint, will lengthen in order to permit that movement to take place. If we have worked them hard or over a long period of time they may remain shorter than the normal resting length. This can create an imbalance between muscles and reduce normal, full-range movement. Have you noticed that on the day following vigorous or unaccustomed sport or exercise your muscles often ache? It can make such a difference to our movement and comfort if we stretch those muscles immediately after exercise.

If we remain sitting for a long time muscles and joints may become set – we become 'chair shaped' - and then feel uncomfortable when we stand up or go to lie down. Regular 'wriggling' and stretching prevents this. Shortened, tight muscles and tendons are far more liable to being strained or torn. This is often just a small, extra reach on an underlying short muscle.

Reduction in length is most obvious in the long muscles which pass over two or more joints.

For example, can you lie on your back, bend your leg, then straighten your knee so your foot faces up towards the ceiling? If so, this shows that your hamstrings are long enough to allow your hip to bend while your knee remains straight. This means you can walk, and run, with a decent stride, bend to pick something off the floor, sit with your legs straight in front of you - or do the Cancan!

While we are growing and our bones are lengthening our muscles sometimes are slower at lengthening (and this may be a cause of "growing pains"). They will gradually stretch as we climb trees, play sport etc. This is one of the many reasons why it is important to be active when we are young and our bodies are developing.

As we age it is quite common to feel stiffer. This may partly be because over the years we have slightly strained some muscle fibres and these have healed with scar-tissue. Or it may simply be that we don't move around so much – too much TV; too long spent at a computer. Whatever the reason I find myself, and so does my husband, and indeed many patients (and even friends who I have bored), that developing a habit of regular, full length stretches is surprisingly helpful at keeping a stiff old age at bay.

When and How to Stretch

- After doing any vigorous activity stretch the muscles you have been using.
- If you hold tension in any group of muscles – usually shoulders, jaw, low back – learn to relax them but also remember to stretch those muscles regularly, and certainly before sleep.
- If you are in one position for any length of time stretch regularly into the opposite position. E.g. if you are weeding in the garden place your hands over your back to support it, and lean backwards.
- Stretch **slowly.** This is because like elastic, if you stretch quickly the muscle rebounds and is activated. (This is useful when we are moving quickly. For example, when we run the quick stretch over the front of the hip stimulates the leg to swing forwards, making it an easier movement.) Once the muscle feels tight, not painful, stay in that position and relax for several seconds. It should not be painful as, of course, we tend to tense up against pain. I think the bigger the muscle the more time it needs. For

example, hold the little jaw muscles on a stretch for about 5 seconds but hold the large thigh muscles for 20-30 seconds.

- Two slow stretches per muscle are probably sufficient. But if you are trying to regain length which you have lost, - it's never too late - do those stretches several times a day, preferably hourly. Usually you can find a convenient position.

- Try taking a few deep breaths once you have reached the tight position. On the breath out the muscle often relaxes and lengthens a little more.

Some people are naturally hyper-mobile – their joints and muscles are very loose. It is usually not advisable for them to stretch as they may overstrain their tissues. Instead they need to tone up/ strengthen their muscles in order to protect their joints.

Individual Stretches

Here are some of the most useful stretches and some different positions to try. Choose the ones most necessary for you and choose the most appropriate position. You may like to do some lying down, because you are in bed, and some during the day while standing or sitting.

Only stretch until the muscle feels tight, not painful, and relax there for several seconds.

Calf muscles:

a) Stand with one foot a good step in front of the other, with both feet pointing forwards, and with your hands resting on a wall in front of you. Keep your back foot flat on the ground and the knee straight. Let your front knee bend until you can feel a stretch down your back leg. Hold that position, relaxing your shoulders and back, and stay there for about 20 seconds. If the tightness goes, you can sneak a bit further.

b) Sit with your heel resting on the floor and your knee straight. Loop a belt, a scarf, or a tie round your toes and pull the foot up towards you until it feels tight down your calf.

c) Stand with the front of your feet on a step; hold on to the banisters; let your heels lower over the edge of the step.

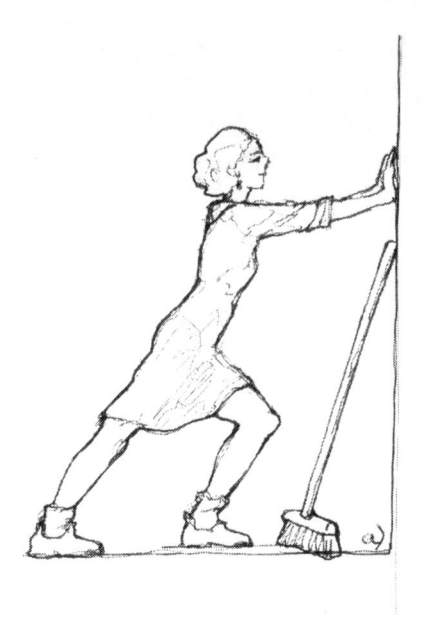

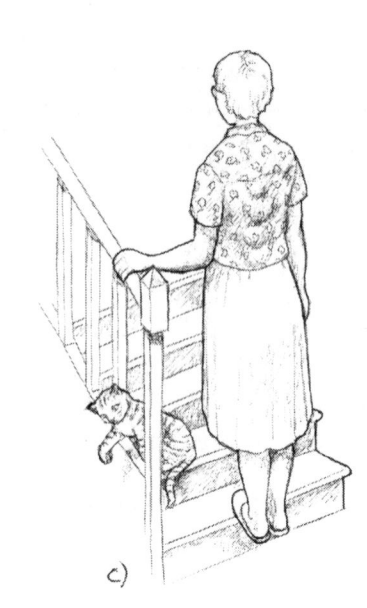

For Plantar fasciitis (see p. 10) – sit with the painful foot resting on the other knee. Hold your toes and pull them and your foot up. This is also a good moment to gently massage the tight tissue.

Thigh muscles – Quadriceps:

a) Lie on your back next to the edge of the bed. Hug one knee up onto your chest – this is to keep your back in a good position. Lower the other leg over the edge of the bed with the knee bent.
b) Lie on your tummy. Bend your knee behind you as far as it will go. You could help it up with the other leg.
c) Stand, holding on if necessary. Bend one knee up in front of you until you can hold your ankle. Then let the leg relax down so that your thigh is alongside the standing leg and you are holding your foot up towards your buttock. If this is too difficult try holding the bottom of your trouser- leg instead of the ankle. Keep your back relaxed; don't let it over-arch.

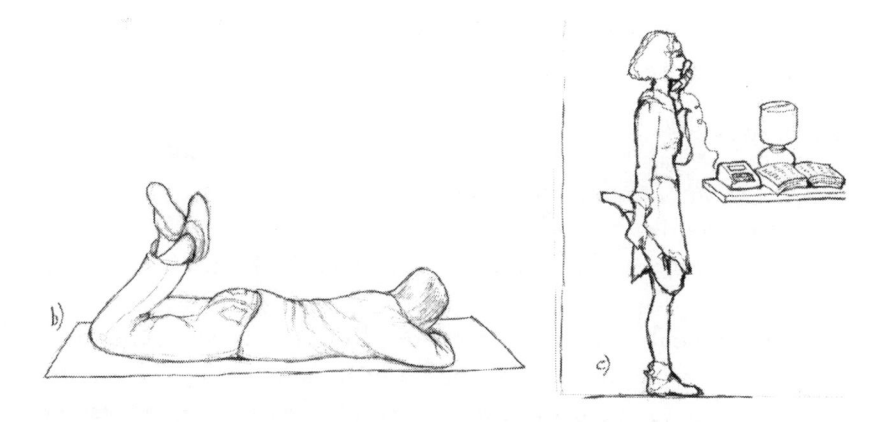

Hamstrings

This is the group of muscles which run down the back of your thigh.
a)   Lie on your back. Bend one leg and place your hands behind your knee with your arms straight and shoulders relaxed. Take your foot up towards the ceiling.

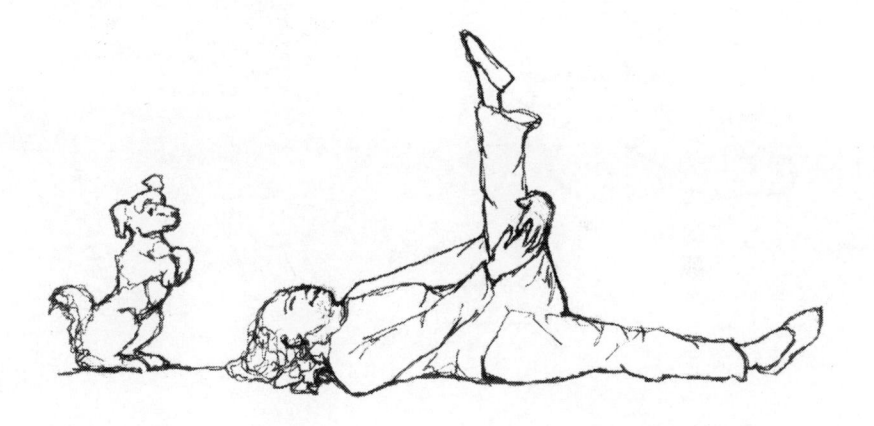

b)   Stand with one foot resting on a convenient step and with the knee straight. Keeping a straight back bow forwards from your hips until you feel a stretch at the back of your thigh.
c)   Stand and gently bend forwards, your fingers towards the floor. Relax in this position, without straining to touch your toes. With a deep breath out you will often find you bend a bit further.

To come up from this position you may prefer to let your knees bend, look up, then straighten up.

Back muscles

a) Lying, standing or sitting: stretch one or both arms above your head, lengthening them.
b) Lie on your back: hug one and then both knees up onto your chest.
c) On your hands and knees: keep your hands where they are and sit back onto your heels. You may find it more comfortable, at first, to sit back onto a pillow which you have placed across your calves. Don't rush this stretch – take a few deep breaths and feel your back relax.
d) Stand with your fingertips over the edge of a sink or low wall; (make sure it is secure). Relax your hips back until your hands, shoulders and hips are level, with your knees straight. Everything should be relaxed except the muscles to your fingers. To come up from this position, bend your knees deeply, look up, and then stand up by straightening your knees.

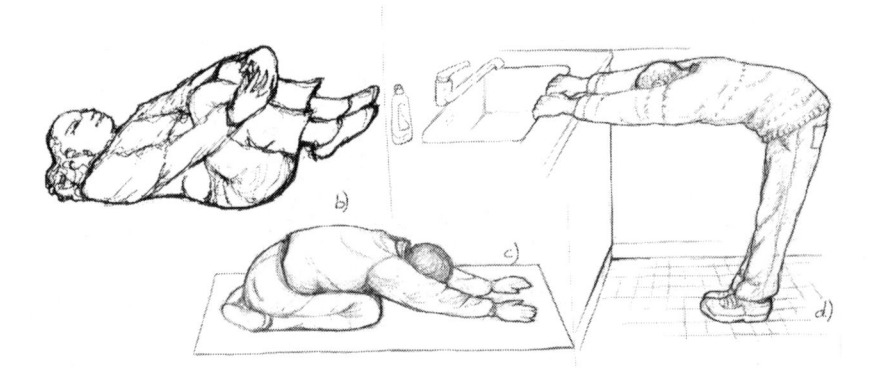

Upper back

a) Lie on your back on a firm surface, with a small pillow under your head and a rolled hand-towel under your upper back. You can place the towel vertically down your spine or horizontally across at the stiffest part. Your knees can be bent or straight. Make sure you are comfortable. You might like to relax in this position for a few minutes.

An Easy Guide to Maintaining a Comfortable (and good looking) Body

To add to the stretch, breathe in and raise your arms above your head; breathe out and let them relax down.

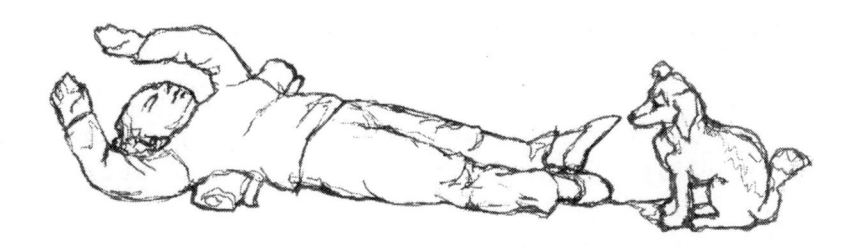

b) Find a firm chair with a back that is level with your shoulder blades. Stretch your arms above your head and lean backwards over the back of the chair. If it is more comfortable, support your head with your hands as you lean back. Keep looking forwards.
c) Sit tall, with your hands behind your head. Lean over to the side with one elbow pointing down and the other up.
d) Sit tall, with hands behind your head. Twist around so that one elbow moves backwards and the other forwards.

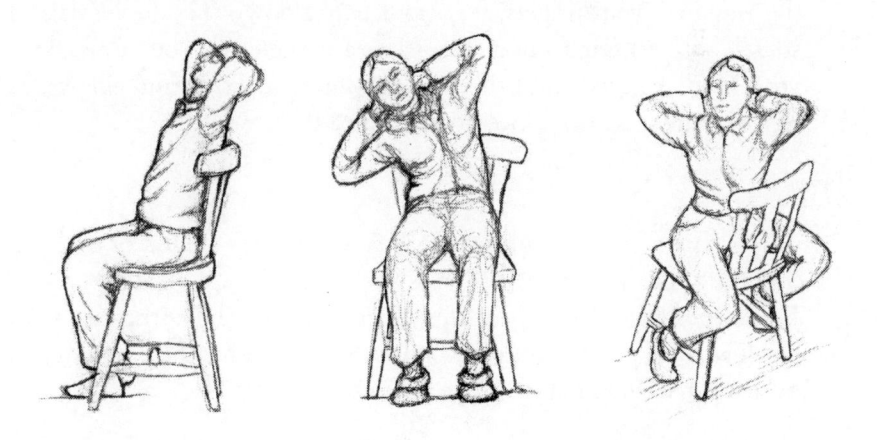

Neck

a) Sit or stand tall: tilt your head sideways, your ear going towards your shoulder. Keep the other shoulder down. Relax and allow the weight of your head to do the stretching.
b) Turn to look behind you.
c) Keeping your chin level and looking straight ahead, draw your head back. This counteracts a tendency for the chin to poke forwards. It is only a small movement but you will feel a stretch at the base of your neck.
d) Let your head relax forwards until you feel a stretch down the back of your neck. You can also take your chin to one side of your chest and then the other and you will feel a slightly different stretch.

Shoulders

The shoulders move in so many directions that there are many different stretches. Here are a few:
a) With your arms beside you, pull both arms down. You will feel a stretch between your neck and shoulders – those stress muscles which often need un-knotting. Also try this with your hands linked behind your back.
b) Sitting, leaning against the back of a firm chair, with your arms hanging beside you: take both arms out and backwards, to stretch the front of your shoulders and chest.
c) Stretch one or both arms above your head.
d) Interlock your fingers, turn your hands down then forwards and stretch both arms in front of you. Pause and then raise your arms above your head. You will find this stretches fingers, wrists and elbows, as well as your shoulders. (See picture on p. 19)

Jaw

This is particularly useful if you grind your teeth at night, or find you are clenching your jaw.

Relax your face. Keep your lips together. Turn the corners of your mouth down and gently pull your chin down. Hold for the count of five and repeat three times before going to sleep.

Forearms

This is useful for those who work at computers or play racquet sports.

a) With your hand facing down straighten your elbow in front of you. Using your other hand gently pull your hand down until you feel a stretch along the back of your forearm. By pulling at a slight angle, to match the direction of the forearm muscles, you will feel a stronger and more effective pull.

b) As a) but pull your wrist and fingers back. Or use stretch d) in Shoulders.

Hands

a) Bend and straighten your fingers.

b) Stretch fingers and thumb apart. Create as much space as possible between your thumbs and index fingers.

Of course there are many other stretches, as you will know if you have done any Yoga. Our bodies are capable of moving in a wonderful variety of ways and feel so much more comfortable if we have maintained that flexibility. I have not included all those positions which stretch rotation, the most complex of movements. But here are a couple to try:

Hip and shoulder rotation

Lie on your back with your knees bent. Place the soles of your feet together and let your knees relax outwards. With your elbows bent to a right angle and arms at shoulder level let your forearms relax backwards. If any part is uncomfortable support it with a pillow.

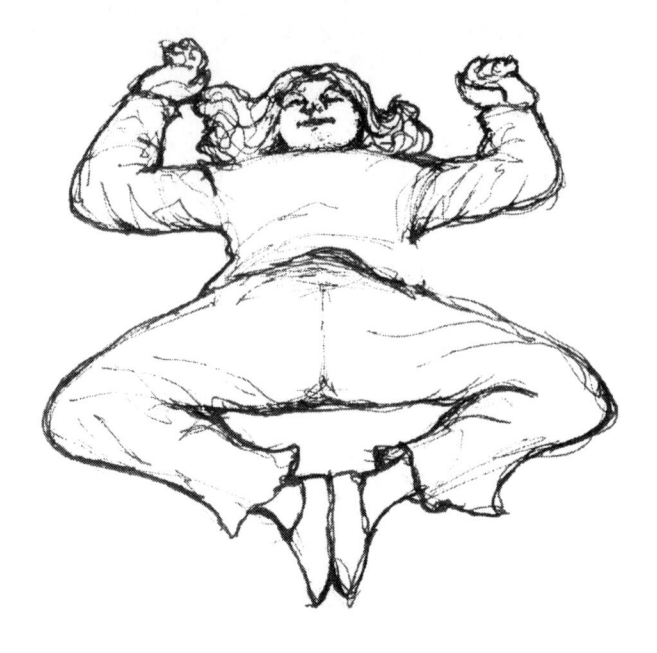

Spinal rotation

Lie on your back with your knees bent and your arms resting out to the side. Let your knees roll over to one side and your head to the other. Relax there for some seconds. Repeat to the other side.

I hope you will quickly get into the habit of stretching regularly - if only for the pleasurable feeling it gives you.

Strength and Control

If we are active in our daily life our muscles will function well and retain their strength. If for any reason we are inactive muscles will gradually weaken. If muscles are weaker we have less support for the weight of our body and therefore postures and movement become more of an effort and more tiring. We may also lose the necessary co-ordination between muscle groups, and this can affect our balance, make us clumsy, and will place unequal stresses on the body.

Each joint has <u>short, deep muscles</u> around it which hold the joint in its correct position and control the fine movements. They work for long periods of time but at a low level, and are designed to do so. If they weaken through lack of use the body has less support.

The deep stomach muscles

Their job is to support the low back and hold the inner organs in place. They don't work when we sit, especially if we slump, and if they weaken the stomach is likely to protrude and the spine sag and shorten. This inflicts extra pressure on the discs and joints of the spine.

The shoulder-blades

Working with them are the little muscles which hold **the shoulder-blades** back. Their job is to maintain the shoulders and upper back in a good position. When functioning correctly the neck and head will balance easily over the rest of the body and the shoulders move freely. If they weaken the shoulders will droop and the chin poke forwards.

To activate these two muscle groups: pull your low tummy muscles in and up, towards your spine. You only need to use about 30% tension. Don't hold your breath or hunch your shoulders. At the same time draw your shoulder-blades back and down, using about 30% tension. This will give you a normal posture and if you get into the habit of doing this whenever you lift something or are in a stooped posture or have to do something awkward, these muscles will support your spine and shoulders. I found that I was unable to lift the heavy anchor of our boat unless I tensioned these muscles, and now I do it for any lifting or heavy carrying – and don't have any back, neck or shoulder problems! I am sure that being aware of this also stopped me having problems when lifting and carrying our two sons when they were little – even when they leapt on me unexpectedly!

Pelvic Floor muscles:

This is a group of muscles that we don't think about at all and yet if they become weak we will have some embarrassing problems. Their job is to support and control the bladder and bowel, so if they become weak there will be some incontinence. Many women think that this is inevitable if you have had children, but men can also have this problem, and usually it can be solved by toning up the muscles. To activate them: pull up the muscles between your legs as though to prevent the passing both of urine and of wind. Hold at about 30% of their full tension for the count of 10. Don't

hold your breath. Can you repeat this ten times? If not they probably need strengthening, which you can do by regular repetitions.
Remember that you can readily tension these small muscles at any time, e.g. when driving, watching TV, walking to work.

Then there are the longer, larger, <u>more superficial muscles</u> which work for shorter bursts and with greater intensity. They should be relaxed when not needed so that they have plenty of stamina for repetitive work.
For example: legs need to walk – think how many steps they need to take each day – so I keep mine strong by walking to and from work and the shops, and enjoy regular longer walks. They need to be able to go up and down stairs, and to push us up out of a chair, so all those are great ways of keeping them strong. Let them swing through easily, when walking, and that way the muscles can relax when not taking your weight. The better your posture the easier they swing.

Of course doing strengthening exercises or going to the gym is a good way to maintain your fitness, but with an active lifestyle you don't have to – unless things go wrong.
It is beyond the scope of this book to describe the many ways of maintaining or improving muscle strength and stamina. My advice, (which I take myself) is to maintain fitness by doing activities you enjoy, as you are far more likely to persist. If you have always been very inactive it is worth trying to do something new; perhaps join a class. You may even find you enjoy it!

<u>Balance</u>

Can you stand on one leg?

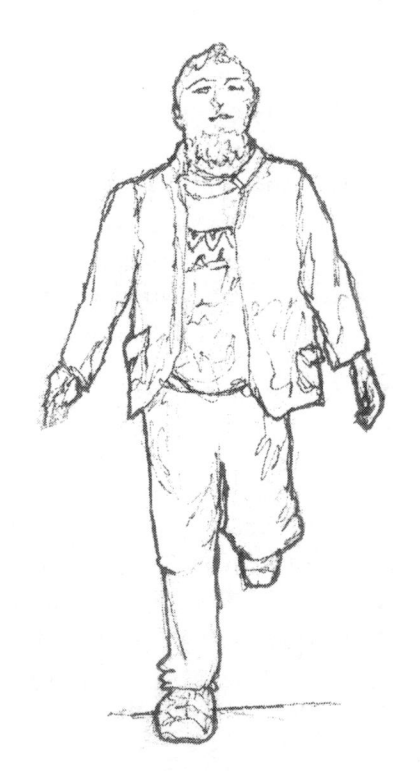

We need to be able to do this so that we can walk with confidence. We have to balance on one leg as the other one swings through. If it is not easy to do this we will tense, walk stiffly, with shorter and wider steps. This imbalance will affect the whole body. When children start to stand and walk they hold their legs apart, and often their arms too, in order to give them better balance but surprisingly quickly they discover the necessary skills to walk more efficiently. As they are constantly active – jumping, climbing, skipping - they practice the necessary skills until they perfect them. The more practice the more skilful. Acrobats can perform amazing balancing acts – with practice. The body must perform many complex things simultaneously to achieve that perfect balance:

- Muscles co-ordinate around the joints – the exact length and amount of contraction to maintain the body in equilibrium.
- There is constant feedback - from the joints, muscles, ligaments, skin, - along the nerves to the brain, informing it where the body is in space and what adjustments need to be made.
- There are complex balance mechanisms in our ears.
- Our eyes check the horizon and our relationship to it. This informs the brain, which gives the necessary orders to keep our alignment. Try balancing with your eyes closed. It is considerably more difficult without that visual information.

As we get older we may lose some of those skills and our sense of balance deteriorates. Is this a natural part of ageing or is it because we don't keep up the practice? Do you perch on the edge of the bed to put on your socks or trousers? Do you find you have to grip the banister as you go up and down stairs? Are you starting to trip over on uneven pavements?

If you have good balance do please maintain it. Once it is lost it can take some persistence to retrain.

If your balance is not good; you feel shaky or nervous standing on one leg, it is well worth regaining it, even though this may take some regular practice. You can save yourself such a lot of trouble. With poor balance you are far more likely to cut or bruise yourself, strain your joints and muscles, drop things, or fall and break a bone. It is also more tiring.

Suggestions: **if your balance is good** – every day when you prepare to put on your socks, stand on one leg, bend down to pick up the sock, put it on. Then do the same with your shoes.

Stand on one leg with your eyes closed. Perhaps you could do it while cleaning your teeth!

If your balance is shaky – stand with your fingertips resting on a surface of a suitable height; fix your eyes on something ahead of you and stand tall; lift up one leg; count to 10. Do this 3 times on each leg. Get into the habit of doing this every time you pass that worktop. Once you are confident doing this, try doing it with less support. Expect it to take many repetitions to gain obvious improvement so keep thinking of the benefits.

Stand on **both** legs, with fingertips resting on a convenient surface. Close your eyes; see if you can count up to ten. Once that is easy, try without touching.

People who do yoga regularly, however old, usually have good balance. This is because they keep practising different balance positions and so maintain those skills.

Chapter 4.
Activities in daily life

<u>In Praise of Walking</u>

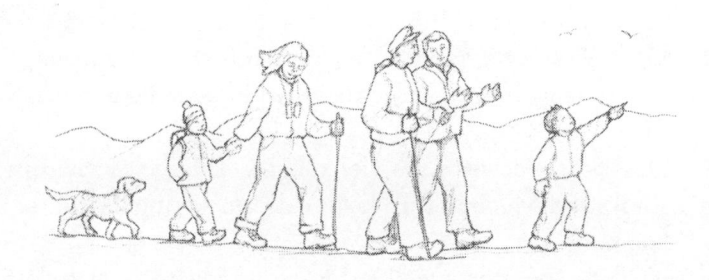

I have always enjoyed walking, which is fortunate as it is one of the best ways of keeping both fit and relaxed. It does all the things that the body needs and in a most natural way. Those of you who already walk regularly have a look at the list of benefits, and congratulate yourself on being so wise. Those of you who don't, have a look and see if you think it would be worthwhile to start.

Benefits of walking:
- √ Weight bearing exercise stimulates bone cells, keeping them strong.
- √ Working the muscles keeps them strong and pliable. It keeps the balance between the strength and length of muscles.
- √ It pumps blood around the body, so all parts are receiving nutrition. Waste products are removed. There is a balance between heat gain and heat loss.
- √ Synovial fluid, the "oil" in the joints, is stimulated, keeping the cartilage in good order and the joints moving smoothly.
- √ Endorphins, the chemicals which help us to relax, are stimulated.
- √ We are inclined to breathe more deeply, especially if going uphill or stepping out faster. Good for our lungs; good for transmission of oxygen throughout the body.
- √ Important for the heart which, being a muscle, benefits from regular extra exercise.
- √ Our inner organs are massaged by the movement, assisting bowel movement.
- √ We look around, moving our eyes and changing focus. This is especially important for those working at a computer with a fixed focus.
- √ Our skin receives ultra-violet light. This helps vitamin D absorption which in turn helps calcium setting. Good for the bones.
- √ It's free - no gym membership required; no special clothes, except perhaps a supportive pair of shoes - and we can go for as long or as short a distance as we like.
- √ With family or friends it is a social occasion. Often the best time to talk.
- √ Exercise like this helps to relieve depression.

I hope you are convinced. If you haven't been walking recently it is wise to start small. Find out how far you can go – and get back – comfortably. Try to do that most days until you are confident that you can manage that distance. Then go just that bit further. Establish that – and then a bit further. You may find your muscles ache at first. Well that's a sign they are working and so getting stronger. But it will become easier and therefore more pleasurable. Keep remembering the benefits!

If you have been for a much longer walk than usual, or on more difficult terrain, stretch your leg muscles immediately after the walk. That will prevent you feeling stiff later on.

Many people find a walking stick is helpful. If you do have a problem leg a stick used in the **opposite** hand will take about 20% of your weight from that leg. If it means you can walk without a limp or a sway that will help the whole body.

Many people like using walking poles – they help to maintain a good rhythm and balance between arms and legs.

A few comments on how to walk:

- **Walk tall.** Think about having a long neck and a long waist. Perhaps it is helpful to remember your helium head and horse's tail! (see p. 35)
- Be relaxed. Check that your back and shoulder muscles are soft.
- Allow your arms and legs to swing through easily.
- Push off with your toes. This is where the power for walking comes from.
- Notice if you tilt or sway to one side. If you do, try to find a level. Imagine you are carrying something on your head. If you are unable to prevent the tilt or sway, use a stick.
- The way you walk will have become your habit so you may not be aware that you stoop or tilt. Notice your reflection in shop windows, or ask your partner to check. Think about leading with your chest rather than your chin.
- As much as possible look around. Don't fix your eyes on the ground all the time or you will begin to stoop – but don't fall into a pothole! Note that it is harder work to lift a leg if your back is bent.
- A dog which tugs on the lead may well cause shoulder problems. Train them not to pull and that will solve the problem. Protect yourself by making sure your shoulder-blade is positioned correctly - back and down

Notice how other people walk – it can be quite an interesting study!

There are many walking groups, catering for all levels, which can be fun to join.

Household Tips

My mother hated housework but loved dancing, and so she always put on music and 'danced' her housework. This works well as when dancing we are lighter on our feet, hold ourselves better, and move rhythmically and easily.

So many of my patients have told me that jobs like hoovering, ironing, washing up, making beds, make their backs ache. Then they tense up, become anxious or frustrated, and the situation gets worse. Sometimes they lose all confidence in their abilities, stop doing these things, and may become depressed. So here are a few tips.

- Try to make sure working surfaces are at a comfortable height for you. Stooping puts greater strain on the spine than standing upright. Arms may complain if the surface is too high.

Set the ironing board correctly for you.

If the sink is too low try having two washing-up bowls and set one on top of the other upturned one. Or perch on a high stool.

- Try putting one foot in front and higher than the other. Often if you open the cupboard under the sink there is a low shelf you can rest your foot on. Or you could rest one foot on a low stool or support of some kind when you are ironing.

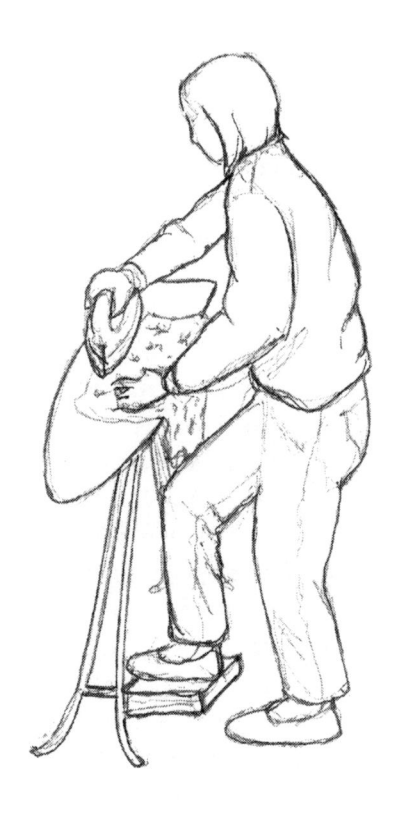

When hoovering try to use your legs by transferring weight from back foot to front foot, rather than making your back do all the work. If you have a hoover with a long hose try holding the hose behind your back. Once you

have got used to this position it is a useful reminder not to lean forwards too much.
- Sometimes it isn't possible to have things at a good height so that is the time to think extra hard about tensioning tummy and shoulder-blade muscles. Bed-making can be really difficult, so **think**.
- Pace yourself. It is so easy to work under pressure - think you must do everything at once, and it must be perfect. Then the body can tense up and begin to ache, or shout "Help. I am in Pain".
Discomfort/pain is usually a message to you saying that it is time to change position and activity. So if you know that hoovering makes your back hurt, for example, only do it for the length of time that it is comfortable; change to some other activity **before** it starts to bother you. Then come back to it at another time. This may well be frustrating at first but very often you will find that because you no longer irritate your back you will gradually be able to increase the time you can do it.

Housework as exercise: All those different activities can be a useful way to keep flexible and fit!

Dusting and polishing, hanging up washing, cleaning windows will exercise your arms and spine.

Lifting saucepans, casseroles, kettles, may maintain some strength but please remember to tension those tummy and shoulder-blade muscles, especially when lifting heavy dishes out of the oven. That will help to keep those muscles strong but also protect your back and shoulders.

Making bread, by hand, keeps your hands wonderfully strong and supple.
Creating cakes etc. is not only satisfying but good work for the arms. Well, that's one excuse…
I am sure you can think of plenty of other activities.
Stretching: reaching for things on a high shelf can be a good way of keeping your arm and back muscles their normal length, but that may be awkward or dangerous, so keep your most frequently used things at a convenient level.

Body Wisdom

> Some exercises you could do while waiting for the kettle to boil.
>
> 1) Think tall and stretch your arms above your head.
> 2) Go up on your toes.
> 3) Stand on one leg and count to ten.

Gardening Tips

Many of the Household tips will apply to work in the garden. I must admit that I get more carried away in the garden and forget how long I've been weeding and planting and pruning, so this is what I try to do:

- Stooping/bending jobs – regularly stand up, place your hands in the small of your back and gently lean backwards.

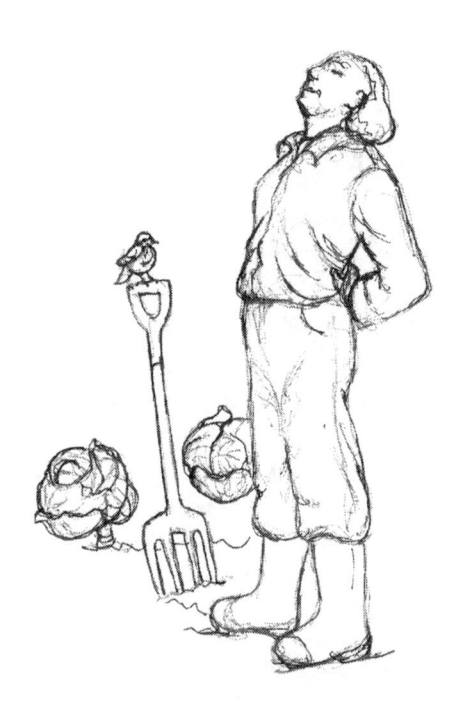

- Always tension your tummy muscles and shoulder-blade muscles when lifting, carrying, straining. Don't over-fill the wheelbarrow or carry weights that are too heavy for you. Two journeys with less weight will be better than one which is a strain.

- When doing repetitive jobs, like potting, make sure you are working at a good height.
- Spring is a busy time. It is like taking up a new sport, or one you haven't played for a while, so go carefully at first, pace yourself. You may well have been less active during the winter and lost some stamina and strength.
- Don't continue an activity which you can feel is giving you trouble. Give it a break. I have treated so many people who have used hedge-cutters or strimmers, in awkward positions, for too long. Then they have to waste time coming to see someone like me.
- Long-handled tools can be helpful.
- A raised bed is not only an efficient way of growing vegetables but easier on the body.
- Stretch your back afterwards – before sitting down for a cuppa.

Driving Tips

Driving is so much a part of most people's lives and yet it is worth being aware that it often causes back, neck and shoulder problems. It is certainly sensible to do whatever you can to prevent these. At least car seats are better designed than they used to be but the first thing to do is make sure yours is adjusted for your comfort and support – not just for anybody else driving the car. Check if it gives you good Lumbar support, that it is tilted correctly so that your neck and shoulders are in good alignment, and that it is the correct distance so that your legs and arms can relax. If necessary add a small cushion for greater back support.

- Sit tall, then position the mirror. When driving don't adjust the mirror if you find you can't see through it, adjust yourself. You have probably slumped.
- Check that your chin is not poking forward. This will strain your neck.
- Check that your shoulder-blades are set back and down. Rounded shoulders will put pressure on joints and tendons. Tense shoulders will compromise the blood supply.
- Wriggle your shoulders up and down every few miles.
- Slide your knees forwards and back regularly. This will lubricate your back. (see p. 2)
- Take breaks if you are driving for several hours, so that you can have a stretch and walk around. This can stop you stiffening up.

- It helps to stretch your back and arms when you arrive.

Occupations

Sedentary jobs e.g. at Computers.

There certainly seem to be more patients coming to physiotherapists with head, neck, back, shoulder and forearm problems since computers have become such common tools. This is not surprising if you consider the bad effects that keeping still have on our circulation, the lubrication of our joints, on our muscles and on our general fitness.

It is unlikely that we will be able to throw away the computer so it seems a sensible idea to work out how we can prevent, or at least limit, all these problems. It is a matter of developing the right habits, so we don't have to think about them, - because of course once we are working at the computer we tend to become absorbed by it.

It is vital to have a good posture, so I am repeating the relevant part from the section on Posture:

Checklist:

- ▶ Is the screen at eye level and straight in front of you? Don't sit on the skew.
- ▶ Is the vision good or do you have to crane your neck forward?
- ▶ Can you get your legs right under the desk so your forearms are supported?
- ▶ Does your chair give you good support? Do you lean away from that supporting back or allow your back to slump? A kneeling-chair will usually place your back in a better position, but you still need to change position regularly or your knees may complain. Or sit on a wedge-shaped cushion so that your thighs are sloping down – or on an Exercise ball. Find out what suits you best; we are all different shapes and sizes.

Even if everything is perfect the body is not designed for this sort of work. Get into the habit of 'wriggling' your shoulders and sliding your knees back and forward. Make sure that every half-hour you get up and walk around or at least have a good stretch. You may need an oven- timer / watch alarm to remind you at first, or a message that flashes up on the screen.

The muscles which we don't use when we are sitting will become weaker.

That will obviously include leg muscles but also stomach muscles and those supporting the shoulder-blades and upper back, though that will depend on your posture. In order to counteract this it is advisable to use your legs as much as possible at other times, do some exercises to tone up the stomach muscles, (there is one easy exercise described in 'Strength and Control'), and develop good postural habits.

Even eye muscles weaken because they are not getting the variety of movement and focus, so be aware of that and look around when walking etc. – or do some eye exercises.

I would strongly advise anyone who spends much time at the computer to take up Yoga or Pilates – or some form of exercise which includes both relaxation and stretching - and to walk regularly.

Hard physical jobs.

Do our bodies wear out faster if we have tough, physical jobs or activities? It seems to me that it is likely that the cartilage which protects joints will become worn, as it does as we age, but that the advantages to the physical body outweigh the disadvantages. Those who do this kind of work are usually stronger, have greater stamina, good lung capacity (as do singers!), and good circulation. All plusses.

However, based on patients I have seen, I think it is worth considering the particular strains on the body in particular occupations, and trying to limit the disadvantages. Here are a few examples and perhaps these suggestions could be applied to similar types of work.

In all cases being over-weight or having a poor posture will place far greater pressure on the body.

In all cases you need to be fit enough for that particular work.

Landscape Gardeners

Repetitive bending of the back, especially if it also involves a twist, puts a great strain on the intervertebral discs. This will be magnified if there is an additional weight e.g. a paving stone. Because discs absorb fluid over-night they are at their 'fattest' in the morning. They are then more vulnerable to pressures which cause them to bulge / prolapse and this can irritate or pinch a nerve. As discs get older they tend to dry out and so become less likely to bulge – one advantage of those extra years – but more pressure may then go onto the joints.

Tips:
- Change your position as often as possible.
- Try to avoid repetitive bending and twisting jobs, especially early in the morning.
- Use your strong leg muscles, tension your tummy muscles and set your shoulder-blades correctly when lifting or doing anything awkward. Don't be pressured into lifting objects that are heavier than you know are safe. (page 37)
- Place your hands over your back and lean backwards frequently, when you are doing a lot of bending. This is sensible and preventative, not a confession of weakness! (see p. 62)
- After work, when your body is tired, avoid sitting in a slumped position. Sit in a chair that gives firm support to the back. Place a cushion in the small of your back if that feels better.
- It can feel really nice to lie flat on the floor for ten minutes or so after work and let the tired muscles relax and stretch out.

Carpet layers.

It's fine to kneel for short periods of time but remaining on your knees for a long time can lead to problems. It puts a lot of pressure through those small knee-caps, and possibly reduces blood flow to your knees by compressing blood vessels in that area. The bursa (a protective pad) at the front of the knee can become inflamed and swollen.

Tips:
- wear knee-pads.
- Stand up frequently and move about – even a few seconds will help.
- Find a couple of minutes to sit, let your legs dangle and give them a good swing. (p. 13)
- Stretch the backs of your legs – Hamstrings and Calves. (p. 47 and 45)
- Stretch your back, which may have been scrunched up in a bent position for too long. (see picture on page 48 and 62)
- Tension your stomach and shoulder-blade muscles when lifting heavy rolls.

Forklift Drivers.

It is often necessary to sit for long periods of time with head, upper back and shoulders in a forward-bend position. This will drag on those areas, causing an over-stretch on the back and a compression on the front of the body. There will be a shearing force on the small joints in the neck and this will eventually damage them. I have seen this leading to nerve damage resulting in severe pain and tingling down the arms and up into the head. This constant position may well become a habit, so that it continues outside of work, which will add to the problem.

Tips:
- Straighten up as often as possible. Think tall.
- Find 'pause' moments to stretch into the opposite position.
- Be aware of your shoulder-blades and set them back.
- After work spend a couple of minutes stretching your neck, shoulders and back.
- Find enjoyable activities outside of work which don't involve sitting.

Carers

You do need to be fit enough for your particular job, so if it is a new type of activity for you it may be sensible to build up your fitness. For example, I have talked with several young women who are carers. They always seem to love the job but are struggling because their backs are aching and they feel they are not going to be able to continue. When they take time off for holidays very often they are pain-free. This is because there is nothing seriously wrong with their backs; they just don't have the muscle strength and stamina yet for a job which entails stooping, often in awkward positions, manoeuvring hoists and wheelchairs, and inevitably some lifting. They would find the work much easier if they were fitter and stronger. They might benefit from going to the gym or a Pilates class or taking up jogging.

Make sure you know how to protect your back when lifting: (see p. 37)

Leisure Activities

Running for Amateurs

Four years ago we started running (well, jogging), hardly ever having done so before. I was 64 and it seemed a good way to give a boost to our ageing hearts and muscles. We started running along a nice, flat beach, but even so I was puffed after about 100 yards. So we alternated running and walking. Gradually the running took over, but any up-gradient was a struggle. We persisted because although each time we thought, "do we really want to do this?" we felt so much better afterwards (and pleased with ourselves!). If we had an ache or two before setting off, it had gone by the time we returned. And our brains seemed sharper too! Now we run for about half an hour at a time, can manage the small hills, and feel so much fitter. It has certainly been worth it.

Running is great for your circulation, improves the strength and stamina of muscles, including the heart muscle, is good for lungs, maintains bone strength. It makes you feel good and can lighten feelings of depression. Recent research suggests that it may stimulate the formation of new brain cells, particularly those involved with memory. That certainly encourages me to keep going!

Tips:
- Don't rush into it. If you have a heart problem check with your GP whether it is advisable.
- Wear shoes which give good support, especially if you have flat feet, and which have good shock-absorbing soles. Avoid high backs on the shoes as these can rub on the Achilles tendon.
- Start small: intersperse running and walking. Gradually lengthen the running time.
- Check your shoulders are relaxed. Your neck may well complain if you hold tension in this area.
- Run smoothly and land softly. Preferably run on grass or paths rather than pavements.
- Do your legs run parallel to each other? Try to avoid your legs swinging out or rolling in.
- Running up hill is of course more difficult. Try changing the length of your stride.
- If you find a section of the run is difficult, occupy your mind. It's amazing how if you are thinking hard about something

else, your legs keep going. You might have a brilliant idea at the same time or sort out a problem.
- Always stretch legs and back after the run, spending 20 seconds on each stretch.
- Remember to have a good glass of water afterwards. Bodies, like plants, suffer from drought.

Cycling.

This is another way of keeping fit and enjoying the countryside. As there is less weight on the legs cycling can be a good choice of exercise if you have problems with your hips or knees.
Make sure the seat and handlebars are the right height for you, so that you are sitting straight and your legs are nearly straight when you push the peddle down. If the handlebars are low, as on racing bikes, you have to tilt your chin up in order to look ahead, and this can cause neck problems.

Swimming and Aqua-aerobics.

Water gives great support to the body. I remember how pleasant it felt to be in the pool when I was heavily pregnant. Swimming and exercising in water is a wonderful way to keep the body flexible. However, if you are anxious about being in water you are likely to tense up so it is probably better to choose another activity.
If you stand with the water half way up your chest this lifts 70% of your weight, so if your have any difficulty with walking this can be a good place to practice. And pushing into the water as you move forwards will strengthen muscles.
Tips:
- If you haven't swum for a while start small. Because it is easier to move in water it is easy to overdo it at first.
- It's advisable to vary the stroke, or do a few exercises in between lengths.
- If you swim with your head out of the water, especially if it is also turned to one side - perhaps chatting with a companion - this can strain the neck, so don't do this for too long. Certainly the spine is in a more natural position if you can duck your face under-water. There is less of a strain in salt water as it gives greater support.

If you have one of those foam 'snakes' try resting your arms over it and letting your body hang down. This gives a delightful stretching feeling to the back.
Hydrotherapy – exercises in a heated pool, initially with professional advice – can be very beneficial if you have any joint or muscle problems.

Dancing / Exercises to music.

The flow and rhythm of music reminds the body to move smoothly, gracefully, joyously. You can dance on your own at home (perhaps while doing the housework) but also enjoy the sociability of going to classes and dances. Complex dance patterns, such as in Scottish dancing, are undoubtedly good for concentration and memory, as well as all the fitness benefits.

Yoga.

As I spend a lot of my working day advising people on suitable exercises I really enjoy going once a week to a yoga class and having someone telling me what to do. Yoga is wonderful for maintaining and improving your posture, flexibility, balance and muscle control. It also teaches you how to relax fully and breathe well.

There are many different forms of exercise and they all have advantages – sports of many kinds, Tai Chi, Pilates, the Alexander technique, Feldenkrais, Keep Fit. If you are interested in exercise find out what suits you, but don't immediately expect to be as good as the teacher. The pleasure is in gradually achieving that.

Chapter 5.
Common Problems

Some of the common problems particular to an area are described in the section about that area. The ones below are more general.

'Aches and Pains'

These can come on gradually or suddenly. Sometimes we can work out why - perhaps something we did the day before - but sometimes they can be quite mysterious, we can't pin them down to any particular strain, and sometimes that can make us anxious that there could be an underlying, sinister cause. Often when patients come to me complaining of an ache I can work out, with a bit of detective work, what the problem is. But sometimes, to be honest, I can't. Fortunately if you follow the recipe below they usually go away. Please note that this does not apply to an area that is hot and inflamed, as this would need a different approach.

- Be kind to it – some warmth, a bit of a rub/a massage.
- Avoid tensing up that area – try to let go/relax it.
- Move it around frequently, but gently, without discomfort. Even very small, soft movements can be beneficial.
- If it seems to be tight or stiff stretch it to the point of tightness and relax there for 10 - 20 seconds. Do this regularly throughout the day.
- Think about why it might have occurred and adjust how you do that activity.

In my experience, with patients and with myself, the ache/pain will go away. It may take a little time but much less time than if you 'protect' it by keeping it still.

Of course if it is a severe pain or it persists then ask advice. There are some conditions which cause persistent, widespread aching and stiffness, which may need medication.

Remember that a feeling of generalised aching throughout the body is often a forerunner to 'flu'.

Arthritis.

This is a much mis-used word. A large number of people who come to me have been diagnosed by their doctor or by themselves with 'Arthritis'. Many of them are understandably anxious because they know someone who indeed has arthritis and is severely disabled.

The word Arthritis means 'Inflammation of joints' – arthro = joint and itis = inflammation. There are various forms of this and it can be a very painful and disabling condition, though now, with advances in pharmacology and surgery, it is much better controlled. There are a number of different forms of arthritis, the most common being Osteo-arthritis and Rheumatoid Arthritis. You will be advised about the management of these conditions by your doctor or physiotherapist. There are several useful books on Arthritis. The advice given below is also relevant.

However, the majority of people do not have that sort of arthritis, even though diagnosed with 'Osteo-arthritis'. Their joints are not inflamed. They have normal degenerative changes in their joints – 'wear and tear', with the cartilage which covers or is between the joints becoming thinner or rougher. Well, that is hardly surprising. You wouldn't expect a machine to keep going without any sign of wear for so many years, - especially if it hasn't been well maintained. Some people may be more genetically liable to these degenerative changes.

What can you do about it? This is the recipe:
- Avoid putting more strain on the joint than is necessary, i.e. lose some weight if you are carrying too much, and try not to carry heavy bags or children.
- Prevent the joints from becoming stiff by plenty of regular mobilising/lubricating exercises. (see 'Lubrication' page 2 or the section on that particular joint). Do some before getting out of bed and when you have been sitting for a while.
- Keep the muscles around the joint strong (or strengthen them)

in order to provide good support and protection for the joint. Keep active.
- Keep the surrounding muscles their correct length by regular stretching.
- Change your position regularly. If you remain still for long it is likely you will stiffen up.
- Think about your posture, especially if the 'wear' is in your neck or back. There will be less force on the joints if you are straight and balanced and relaxed.
- If the problem is in your legs wear a good pair of shoes which prevent your feet rolling in.
- Avoid walking with a sway, as this will put a shearing force onto your hips, knees and ankles. Use a stick if necessary – until you can eliminate the sway.
- Joints often like some warmth. – it helps to improve the circulation and to relax the surrounding muscles. If the joint is swollen it may prefer an ice-pack.

A lady in her late sixties came to me with a painful, stiff hip which was making many of her normal activities difficult. X-ray showed that she had degenerative changes in the joint and it was suggested that she might need a hip replacement. She followed the recipe above and regained quite a lot of movement in the joint. She was able to increase the distance she could walk comfortably and do all her household activities. As long as she did a few exercises before getting out of bed she was able to get her socks on. Most importantly the pain was so much better she felt she could put off surgery. She may need a hip replacement in the future, but she is happy to delay this.

Wheatbags give a very soothing warmth, so if you have a microwave you could buy or make yourself one.

> **How to make a wheatbag:**
> Using some cotton sew a bag about 9 inches long and 3 inches wide. Before you sew up the fourth side fill it about ¾ full with any grain – wheat, rice, barley. Sew up the last side, and you are ready to heat it in the microwave for approx. one minute. In fact you can make it any shape or size (or colour) you like but this size lies comfortably over most joints.
> Of course you can use other forms of warmth. If it is a hot-water-bottle place it in a cover or wrap it in a towel. Too much heat could damage the skin.

Illness

If you are in bed for any length of time it is usually wise to move around gently and regularly. When you are recovering it may take some time to get back to your normal activities, neither being too fearful of movement nor too hasty to push your body before it has regained some strength and stamina. Gradually, over some days or weeks, extending the distance you can walk is often the best way to recover. You may be given specific advice and exercises to help rectify your particular problem.

Injury

Injuries such as broken bones, torn muscles and tendons take a certain length of time to heal. If this is a severe injury you will have been to hospital or visited your GP and will have been given treatment and advice for that particular injury, so I will only make some general points.

Broken bones:

These usually require some form of fixation and will require several weeks to heal, depending on the size of bone and your age. Children's bones knit together more quickly than those of adults - in fact in about half the time. The surrounding muscles will weaken because of the enforced inactivity so that when the fixation is removed (usually plaster), people are often horrified how uncomfortable and weak that part feels, when they thought they would be completely better. Well, the bone is healed and now you must regain mobility and strength, which may well take some persistence.

Aim for 100% recovery, as you are less likely to have future problems if you are fully mobile and strong. This could take some weeks of regular exercising and stretching. If it has not been possible to set the bone exactly, it is not always possible to regain full mobility – but it is certainly worth a try. While in plaster keep the rest of the body moving well, especially neighbouring joints and muscles. This improves the circulation, which assists the healing process, and will also help to maintain strength. You can even encourage some useful muscle strength inside the plaster by tensioning and relaxing those muscles, comfortably and regularly.

Torn muscles:

The belly of a muscle has a very good blood supply, so if some of the fibres tear it may bruise quite dramatically. The good thing is that, with that good supply, they heal faster. It still takes some time, depending on the severity of the tear, and it will heal with some scar-tissue. You will need to gradually regain its normal length, by careful and regular stretching, and its strength, by repetitive exercise and activity. Be advised when and how to start doing this.

Torn or sprained tendons and ligaments:

These structures have poor blood supplies and so can be quite slow to repair. Boost the circulation by regular, pain-free movement. Even very small movements can be effective. Local massage, which you can do yourself, can help too. Of course if the tear is a severe one get advice about how much you should, or should not, move the part.
Immediately after injury it is likely that that area will be swollen, perhaps bruised. It can speed recovery if you can reduce the swelling by using an ice-pack, a supporting bandage, and are able to keep that part raised, above the level of the heart, for as long as is practical, during the first couple of days. This can be a good position in which to do some appropriate exercises.

Breathlessness.

This book should not be used as a textbook for those with chest problems. However there are a few simple guidelines on breathing which may be useful.
A feeling of breathlessness is a frequent symptom of any chest condition but also occurs with panic attacks and stress. It can be quite frightening

and the overwhelming feeling is the need to get more air into the lungs. And so the tendency is to start breathing in very rapidly – but to no good effect. The reason for that is that once you have taken a breath in the lungs are filled. You need instead to breathe **out,** emptying the lungs of that stale air. Then you will automatically breathe in fresh air. This may take a little practice at first, so my 3 tips for anyone with these problems are:

- Learn how to relax (see p. 41/42) being particularly aware of your shoulder girdle.
- Learn to understand your lungs and how to use them fully. Note that lungs are triangular in shape, with the point of the triangle near the collarbone, so most benefit will come from using the base of the triangle i.e. the lower and wider part of the lungs. Learn to be able to control your breathing. (see p. 41)
- Keep your spine and rib-cage flexible.

The more familiar you are with these three tips the more you will be able to reduce breathlessness and improve your lung function. Ask for help and advice from a specialist physiotherapist or nurse if you need it.

Chapter 6.
Keeping Old Age at Bay

As I walk along the street I see so many older people who are stooped. Worryingly I am seeing more of my friends looking at the ground, their heads and shoulders forward as they walk, and somehow shorter than they used to be. I sometimes wonder if this isn't the fault of those road signs near Homes alerting us to old people crossing, showing a stooped couple. Or perhaps it is our sensitive brains picking up other people's posture and responding to that peer-group pressure. I long to tell them how dangerous it is to give way to this stoop; how once gravity gets on your back it will push you down, physically and perhaps psychologically too. It is not necessary; it is much more fatiguing; it throws the whole co-ordination of the body out of kilter; it can all too quickly become a habit. **Please think tall!**

Some of this problem may be due to deteriorating balance and therefore loss of confidence. So do **practice your balance**. Keep active so that muscles remain strong and circulation good. If an illness has set you back, gradually get back to your previous level of activity. It's worth the effort.

Remember how easy and how valuable it is to **'wriggle'** – keeping the joints oiled. If you find that you feel stiff in the morning, that couple of minutes spent gently moving about before you get up is invaluable. You should find that you can get your socks on more easily if you have gently hugged your knees up onto your chest a few times or sat on the edge of the bed and bent down a few times.

Soft tissue – muscles, ligaments, connective tissue – may stiffen with age. There may be some scarring within the tissue. If we habitually **stretch,** in those pause moments – waiting for the eggs to boil, looking out of the window, while watching TV or listening to the radio, – this will lessen that stiffening and keep us moving with greater ease. We may have to accept some discomfort or loss of movement, as the body doesn't renew itself so efficiently as we age, but we can without doubt limit this by keeping active. I believe this simple maintenance work makes an enormous difference to the comfort of our bodies as we get older. It is not miraculous but I have been in the position to compare those who do and those who don't.

Oh, and find every opportunity to laugh! It is a great way to release those lovely chemicals, the Endorphins.

Danger – Beware!

Robert used to work in an office, sitting all day, but he walked briskly to and from the station and at weekends would go for longer walks and play tennis with his family. When he retired he continued to walk but perhaps not daily. Then he had a couple of short stays in hospital and slowed down further. He sat slumped over the newspaper or watching TV. He began to say "I'm getting old. No, I can't be bothered to go out."

Does this sound familiar to you?

Robert began to find it difficult to go upstairs, his legs protesting, feeling breathless. He installed a stair-lift. With weaker legs and trunk his balance became shaky and he started to lose confidence, feel tired, had no energy and became depressed. As his pelvic floor muscle weakened he kept having to go to the toilet and then needed to wear pads. Normal daily activities became a struggle and his wife had to do more and more for him. She became tied to his requests, then demands, for assistance. His sleep, and then hers, became disturbed; by now he was fearful of getting up on his own – and he needed to get up several times in the night.

What will happen when his legs have lost so much strength that he is unable to get up from his chair?

However, with medication, he could well live another 10 – 20 years. We rejoice in our longevity but not if we have lost all quality of life.

What makes me sad, even angry, about this not uncommon tale is that it need not have happened. Unnecessarily two peoples' lives have been destroyed by Robert's failure to act. Beware! Don't let this happen to you. It just takes some regular activity to maintain strength and some will-power to build up that activity again if there has been a setback. This may not be easy at first but the consequences of not doing so can be devastating.

Summing up

If you have read all of this it may seem as though we have to be thinking about our body all the time. Who wants to do that! But if we can get into a few easy habits, so that they become automatic, this can be very effective and once established won't take much thought or time.

"Prevention **is** much better than cure", so if you are young and lead an active life, keep it up, enjoy it, don't feel that you haven't time for activities – they will save time in the long run.

If your job keeps you active that is fine. Just make sure you know how to lift, how to manage repetitive actions safely, develop the habit of stretching regularly - and know how to relax.

If you spend most of the time sitting or standing still your muscles will tend to become weaker and shorter. It pays to spend time, outside of work or travelling to and from work, working those muscles. But not just at weekends. Many people sit all week and then perhaps garden vigorously all weekend – and are surprised that they suffer for it.

It is so sensible to have a good posture at work, so think how you can make that easy for yourself. And stretch regularly into an opposite posture. It's a useful moment to pause and think

Just because you are getting older don't become less active. You may prefer to modify your chosen activity if it has been very competitive and your body is complaining. Walking, cycling, swimming etc. rather than football, for example. Walking to the shops, doing housework, gardening can all help.

Avoid staying in one position for long.

Why bother? Well everyday life is much easier and pleasanter if you are fit, flexible and comfortable. You are likely to recover from illness and injury more quickly if your body works well. If it has stiffened, lost stamina or the ability to balance, everything becomes much more of an effort, less comfortable and risky - as tissues are more easily damaged.

"If you don't use it you lose it". Indeed it is easier to maintain strength and stamina than regain it - but it is never too late to improve.

Whatever your age you will feel good, look good and reduce future problems if you develop these few easy habits:

Body Wisdom

**Relax. 'Wriggle'. Stretch.
Be aware of posture. Keep active. And enjoy it.**

Suggested Daily Routine

Before getting out of bed gently move about, especially any area you know feels stiff. Do a few exercises.

Throughout the day be aware of your posture. Think tall.

Get into the habit of using 'pause' moments to stretch.

Practice your balance, whether to maintain or improve it.

Don't remain in the same position, without moving, for longer than half an hour. Move around, wriggle, stretch, smile.

Be aware of unnecessary muscle tension. Learn how to relax.

Think how to protect your body when doing heavy or repetitive work – correct positioning, tensioning supporting muscles.

Take some extra exercise, appropriate to your situation. If you can walk, go for a walk.

About The Author

Physiotherapy can be a wonderfully satisfying and varied career. Jackie Wright, MCSP, MACP, has made good use of the opportunities. She has worked for the National Health Service - in hospitals, clinics and in the community - but also in Uganda, Italy, Australia and Malawi. She has taught in a School of Physiotherapy and spent two years with VSO (Voluntary Service Overseas) helping to establish a Rehabilitation Training School.

It hasn't all been work. She travelled by land-rover from England to Southern Africa and many years later she sailed with her husband and two sons from Australia.

Most recently she has been working in Woodbridge, Suffolk, where she now lives.

Sandra Morris is an artist and English teacher and has also lived in many parts of the world. She and Jackie are cousins.

Lightning Source UK Ltd.
Milton Keynes UK
16 February 2011

167628UK00002B/227/P